Master the Healing Art of Foot Reflexology

A Workbook

written by Susan Watson

illustrated by John Gibbs and Nancy Erickson

Disclaimer: This workbook is for informational purposes only; this is not a substitute for medical diagnosis. Before embarking on this program, if you or your client has a serious illness, it is highly recommended speaking with a medical doctor and telling him or her your plans with reflexology. Do not stop taking any medication before consulting your physician.

First printing, May 2003

ISBN: 0-9719437-0-2

Printed in the United States of America
BookMasters, Inc.

Forward

Reflexology is a gift everyone should give and receive. It is a present that will last a life time. Praise goes to my friend Susan Watson who wrote this book which teaches reflexology in a very simplified manner. The book is easy to follow and "it's simple to understand the concepts." Reflexology is an ancient art which is fun to learn and the effects are almost magical. When the endorphins (the body's own natural pain medication) are flowing through the body after one single treatment you will be amazed that you were able to learn this wonderful simplified technique by reading "Master the Healing Art of Foot Reflexology". I highly recommend this book for anyone who wants to feel better and help others feel good.

Dr. Shelly Soble, D.P.M.
Podiatrist and Medical Reflexologist

Special Thank Yous

Thank You to my husband, Greg, who lovingly supported me through this book.

Thank You to Nancy Erickson for all her wonderfully detailed artwork.

Thank You to Alan Bonness for his work with the graphic design on the book cover design and foot charts.

Thank You Lorraine Graham and Addi Faerber for taking pictures.

Thank You Wilma Faerber, Bonnie Staas, and Karen Meadows for the proofreading.

Thank You to Rick Faerber, Gary Graham, Terry Vecchio, and Sara Bonness for being my foot models.

Thank You John Gibbs for changing my photos to drawings.

Thank You to Northern Prairie, a Center for Education and Healing Arts in Sycamore, Illinois. If it was not for them asking me to teach Reflexology, I may not have written this Workbook.

Thank You to Ed Mikkelson for your advice in layout and typesetting.

My Story

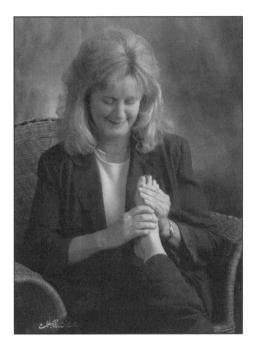

My interest in Reflexology began in the 1960's when my mother mentioned to her sister and brother-in-law, Marjorie and Elbert Hubbs, that I was having a bed-wetting problem at the age of 12. My uncle, who was a reflexologist, and trained by Eunice Ingham, immediately began to manipulate pressure points on my feet. I remember it was painful in certain areas, and they would tell me, "that is your kidney area. We need to work out this pain to help your kidney". I also felt a feeling of well-being come over me that I will never forget. They taught me which area to press, and within a few short weeks the problem disappeared.

I remembered the stories my uncle and aunt told me how they had helped many people with so many problems. I had another aunt, Dorothy Gallaher who also inspired me. Aunt Dorothy was also a reflexologist, trained by Eunice Ingham and Mildred Carter. She, too, had many stories to share about all the people she had helped to heal. From that time on, I wanted to be like them -- a Reflexologist.

- Certified by the International Institute of Reflexology, in St. Petersburg, Florida

- Nationally Board Certified through the ARCB (American Reflexology Certification Board)

- Certified practitioner by "Father Josef method of Reflexology"

- Certified member of the Reflexology Association of Illinois

- Advanced training taught by Dr. Jesus Manzanares

It has been a wonderfully gratifying job, helping people feel better!

Suggested Reading List

Dwight Byers- Better Health with Foot Reflexology- Anatomy & Reflexology Helper Areas

Eunice Ingham- Stories the Feet Can Tell & Stories the Feet Have Told

Mildred Carter- Helping Yourself with Foot Reflexology- Body Reflexology

Kevin & Barbara Kunz- The Practitioner's Guide to Reflexology- Feet Don't Lie

Christine Issel- Reflexology: Art, Science, and History

Beryl Crane- Reflexology: The Definitive Practitioner's Manual

Laura Norman- Feet First

Hanne Marquardt- Reflex Zone Therapy of the Feet

Ann Gillanders- The Ancient Answer to Modern Ailments

This is just a few books, as there are at least fifty books published on Reflexology.

Suggested Web Sites on the Internet

www.thumbwalking.com

www.reflexology-research.com

www.pacificreflexology.com

www.reflexologyworld.com

www.reflexology-usa.org

www.foot-reflexologist.com/EGYPT_1.HTM

www.reflexology.org

If interested in schools of Reflexology go into your favorite Internet search engine and type Reflexology schools, and a list will come up. The International Institute of Reflexology has seminars across the U.S.

Testimonials

Since I have started reflexology treatments on a regular basis with Sue Watson, I have an overall sense of well being and health. I feel a sense of vibrancy after a session. On several occasions I have had a stiff neck and the treatment immediately gave relief to the neck area. I have also had congestion in the chest area and after not being able to breathe properly for days had relief with one treatment. Reflexology has also given me IMMEDIATE relief from headaches.

Sandy Carmichael, Owner
Options 4 Health

Sue Watson has worked wonders in my life. I have weekly reflexology treatments and my health has totally turned around. I no longer have to take my blood pressure pills. I used to live on every type of acid reducer pill available and have almost totally eliminated having to take anything for what was a chronic problem I have lived with for 30 years. I also had been taking drops for glaucoma and when I went to the eye doctor last month- he said my glaucoma has virtually disappeared. I no longer need those drops. Reflexology and Sue Watson have given me a new lease on life!

Jim Carmichael, Owner
Carmichael Construction, Inc.

Reflexology, through skilled thumb and fingers, flies to the pain core bringing instant relief. It can heal and keep you agile without medicines. As a emphysema patient it immensely improved my physical strength. It also helped my arthritis, made me relax and feel like I was walking on air.

Anna Belle Nimmo
Freeport, IL.

I was suffering with vertigo caused by an inner ear viral that had me in a tail spin. After seeing two doctors and losing a week of work not being able to focus on anything, I was told it had to run its course. In the mean time a friend suggested that I see Sue. Sue located through my feet the problem in the inner ear, but much to my surprise she found another problem I've had to live with. suffered with an ongoing kidney problem for the past several years, feeling the need too constantly used the rest room. After being treated by doctors with many different medications, the symptoms would always return, so after the years I have learned to live with it. After a few visits with Sue I no longer feel the sensation of having to frequent the facility. Currently I am a regular customer of Sue's, not only does she keep me feeling healthy with good circulation, I feel a surge of energy after a session and that is a delight when a busy lifestyle requires so much motivation in a single day.

Thank You, Sue.
Teri Volpentesta

I have had heel pain for years. It would come and then go.
One time it came and would not leave. I was miserable.
I went to my physician and he gave me pills. They did not work.
I went to the chiropractor and he could not help me.
I went to the foot doctor and he did not help me.
Then I heard about a lady named Sue who did reflexology. She literally pushed the pain out of my feet. I went on a treatment schedule with her and the pain is gone.
If the pain comes back I will look to reflexology.

Steven T. Turner

I had Sue's phone number for almost a year before meeting her. We met at a holistic health fair and after a half hour treatment I knew my feet/body needed more work. Due to the effects of sugar diabetes I had very little feeling in my left foot. Also, my back and hips often bothered me after getting up in the morning. After a few weekly visits from Sue, my foot is very much improved and I only have numbness in it occasionally, which corrects itself in a short time. My back and hips are less painful and I have been able to cut down on taking so many pills for pain management. Reflexology has helped me very much.

Linda Meadows

I had been experiencing a problem with my right hand. It was the start of carpal tunnel I was told. Most of the time my hand felt like it was asleep and I had trouble grasping and holding on to things. I ran across Sue Watson and asked her if she could do anything for hands. I knew she did reflexology on feet but unsure if she did hands. So, I let Sue work on my right hand. She did one treatment and it hurt! The next day my hand started to feel better. In two days I could grasp and hold objects. That was two years ago. I have not had a problem with my hand since.

My next session with Sue was when I experienced sciatica on my right side. I gave Sue a call and made the appointment and Sue worked on both feet. The next day the pain was less. In three days no signs of pain. I believe in reflexology. Sue knew when she was working my feet that I had a problem with my left kidney. My doctor had told me recently that my kidneys were not working properly. Sue knew which kidney was causing me difficulty and is having me work on that area of my foot everyday. I will not know my results until   my next doctor appointment, but I feel that Sue's treatment will make a difference.

I would recommend reflexology to anyone.

Sincerely,
Janet Wise

Sue is a wonderful healer and caring practitioner. Although I was not aware what exactly was "off-kilter" in my body, Sue was able to find those tender, congested places that needed to be worked out. Reflexology is an old healing tradition that will find new followers under Sue's teaching with this book.

Karen Meadows

Sue has been working on my feet for quite sometime. I have a heel spur and my entire foot hurt when she started. There was shooting pain going up the back of my heel, but not anymore. My arch was very painful. Her massage is wonderful. I'm not sure what caused the spur, perhaps improper walking over a long period of time, but she works out the inflammation. There are many nerve endings on the bottom of the feet and they need to be relaxed and free of inflammation, she works on all of the areas.

Maxine Kahler

Note:

This workbook is designed as an educational tool for better health. Reflex areas and information are included as examples to help you learn. They are not diagnostic or prescriptive.

Everyone's needs are different. I encourage you to listen to your own body, and complement this information with the advice of a qualified health professional.

This is brief anatomy. For further information I recommend Grays Anatomy.

Disclaimer: This workbook is for informational purposes only; this is not a substitute for medical diagnosis. Before embarking on this program, if you or your client has a serious illness, it is highly recommended speaking with a medical doctor and telling him or her your plans with reflexology.

Do not stop taking any medication before consulting your physician.

"The art of medicine consist of amusing the Patient, while nature cures diseases." -Voltaire

Preventative Therapy--
Ten Minutes a Day for Health

Circulation is the key to good health. Your blood has to get to all parts of the body if it is to remove the poisons that are secreted by each and every cell, and to remove the many dead cells. In today's world we do not get enough exercise. There is no substitute for regular exercise and good eating habits.

If you take it upon yourself to exercise your organs, glands, and systems of the body through reflexology once a day, this will help to circulate your blood to each system of the body. You should develop a habit to work on yourself ten minutes each day.

Sit down and put your feet, one at a time, up on your lap, then thumb-walk or massage each and every reflex area, as described through this book. Pay attention to the sensitive areas. These may be future trouble spots, and will need more attention for healing to occur.

Using reflexology techniques will help to relieve stress and tension throughout your body.

Good luck, and happy reflexing!

Table of Contents

Chapter 1- About Reflexology

What is Reflexology and what are the benefits? 3
History of Reflexology 4-6
Possible reactions to a Reflexology session 7
Reflexology Rules/ When not to use Reflexology. 8
Research Studies done on Reflexology 9
Frequently Asked Questions 10-11
What does "Sensitivity Spots" Mean? 12
Can I use Reflexology on Children? 13-14
Can I use Reflexology on the Elderly? 15
Can I use Reflexology on Cancer Patients? 16-17
Can I use Reflexology on someone who is Pregnant? 18

Chapter 2- Anatomy/Guidelines/Zones of the Foot

Anatomy of the Bones of the Foot 21
Diagram of the Bones of the Foot. 22
Front View of Foot Muscles 23
Back View of Foot Muscles. 24
Side View of Foot Muscles and Tendons 25
Terms of Anatomical Direction. 26-27
Biomechanics of the foot. 28-31
Guidelines of the Foot 32
Locating the Zones of the Foot. 33
The Meridian Theroy 34
Referral Areas. 35
Quiz on Anatomy of the foot. 36

Chapter 3 - Holding & Thumb Walking Techniques   39-41

Chapter 4 - Relaxing Techniques   45-47

Chapter 5 - Central Nervous System, Reflex Points, and their Disorders

Basic Anatomy of the Central Nervous System. 51-56
Locate the reflex areas of the Central Nervous System 57
Answer key to the reflex location of the Central Nervous System . . . 58-59
How the work the Central Nervous System reflex areas 60-63
Central Nervous System Disorders and the helper reflexes . . 64-76
Quiz on the Central Nervous System 77

Table of Contents

Chapter 6- Sense Organs, Reflex points, and their Disorders

Basic Anatomy of the Sense Organs. 81-84
Locate the reflex areas of the Sense Organs 85
Answer key to the reflex location of the Sense Organs 86
How to work the Sense Organ reflex areas 87
Sense Organs Disorders and the helper reflexes 88-99
Quiz on the Sense Organs 100

Chapter 7- Endocrine System, Reflex Points, and their Disorders

Basic Anatomy of the Endocrine System. 103-108
Locate the reflex areas of the Endocrine System. 109
Answer key to the reflex location of the Endocrine System . . . 110-111
How the work the Endocrine System reflex areas. 112-114
Endocrine System Disorders and the helper reflex areas . . 115-125
Quiz on the Endocrine System 126

Chapter 8- Circulatory System, Reflex Points, and their Disorders

Basic Anatomy of the Circulatory System 129-130
Locate the reflex areas of the Heart 131
Answer key to the reflex location of the Heart 132
How to work the Heart reflex areas 133
Heart Disorders and the helper reflex areas 134-142
Quiz on the Circulatory System 143

Chapter 9- Digestive System, Reflex Points, and their Disorders

Basic Anatomy of the Digestive System 147-150
Locate the reflex areas of the Digestive System 151
Answer key to the reflex location of the Digestive System . 152-153
How to work the Digestive System reflex areas 154-159
Digestive System Disorders and the helper reflex areas. . . 160-183
Quiz on the Digestive System. 184

Chapter 10- Urinary System, Reflex Points, and their Disorders

Basic Anatomy of the Urinary System 187-188
Locate the reflex areas of the Urinary System 189
Answer key to the reflex location of the Urinary System 190
How to work the Urinary System reflex areas 191
Urinary System Disorders and the helper reflex areas 192-200
Quiz on the Urinary System 201

Table of Contents

Chapter 11- Respiratory System, Reflex Points, and their Disorders

Basic Anatomy of the Respiratory System 205-208
Locate the reflex areas of the Respiratory System. 209
Answer key to the reflex location of the Respiratory System. . . 210
How to work the Respiratory System reflex areas. 211-212
Respiratory System Disorders and the helper reflex areas. 213-223
Quiz on the Respiratory System. 224

Chapter 12- Lymphatic System, Reflex Points, and their Disorders

Basic Anatomy of the Lymphatic System. 227-228
Locate the reflex areas of the Lymphatic System. 229
Answer key to the reflex location of the Lymphatic System. . . . 230
How to work the Lymphatic System reflex areas. 231-232
Lymphatic System Disorders and the helper reflex areas . . 233-237
Quiz on the Lymphatic System. 238

Chapter 13- Hip/Knee/Leg/Shoulder, Reflex Points, and their Disorders

Basic Anatomy of the Hip, Knee, Leg, Shoulder, Elbow, and Wrist .
. . . . 241-243
Locate the reflex areas of the Hip, Knee, Leg, Shoulder, ...
Elbow, and Wrist. 244
Answer key to the reflex location of the Hip, Knee, Leg, ...
Shoulder, Elbow, and Wrist. 245
How to work the Hip, Knee, Shoulder, Elbow, ...
and Wrist reflex areas 246-247
Hip, Knee, Leg, Shoulder, Elbow, and Wrist Disorders and the . . . .
helper reflex areas. 248-251
Quiz on the Hip, Knee, Leg, Shoulder, Elbow, and Wrist 252

Chapter 14- Reproductive System, Reflex Points, and their Disorders

Basic Anatomy of the Reproductive System 255-257
Locate the reflex areas of the Reproductive System 258
Answer key to the reflex location of the Reproductive System . . 259-260
How to work the Reproductive System reflex areas 261-262
Female Reproductive Disorders and the helper reflex areas. . . . 263-274
Male Reproductive Disorders and the helper reflex areas . 275-279
Quiz on the Reproductive System 280

Table of Contents

Chapter 15- The Skin, Reflex Points, and their Disorders

Basic Anatomy of the Skin Organ and How to work the . . . .
Skin reflex areas 283
Locate the reflex areas of the Largest Organ of the body, ...
the Skin 284
Skin Disorders and the helper reflex areas 285-290
Quiz on the Skin Anatomy 291

Chapter 16- Foot Ailments

Pathologies of the Foot 295-296
Foot Ailments 297-298
How to work Foot Ailments 299-302

Chapter 17- Sample Reflexology Session

Sample Reflexology Session 305-307
Stretch you hands between clients 308

Chapter 18- Marketing Yourself, Clients History Forms, and Documenting the Charts of Your Clients

How to Market Yourself 311
Sample Client History Form 312
Sample Documenting Form 313

Chapter 19- Foot Charts

Right Foot 317
Left Foot 318
Top of Foot 321
Side of Foot 322
Answer Key to the Quizzes 325

Answer Key to the Quizzes
325

1 Chapter

About
Reflexology

What is Reflexology?

Reflexology is a science that deals with the principle that there are over 7,200 nerve endings on each foot. These nerve endings connect to nerve pathways that lead to each and every organ, gland, and part of the body.

Through the use of a unique thumb and finger walking technique on each foot, sensory nerves carry information to the brain and help release endorphins to reduce pain in the body. The theory is that crystal deposits form at the nerve endings, this keeps the electrical impulses of the nerves from grounding. By breaking up the crystal deposits in the feet the crystals are carried off into the blood stream and eliminated through the urinary system. This relieves the congestion in the body and the body functions flow smoothly.

Reflexology brings the body into homeostasis (a balancing of the endocrine glands) and is capable of improving the function of all body systems, while leaving you with a feeling of harmony and balance.

What are the Benefits of Reflexology?

- Reflexology reduces stress, tension, and anxiety
- Reflexology increases blood and lymphatic flow
- Reflexology improves oxygen and nerve supply
- Reflexology normalizes glandular function
- Reflexology cleanses the body of toxins
- Reflexology balances all body's systems
- Reflexology improves emotional imbalances
- Reflexology is a preventative health care
- Reflexology enhances a massage and a chiropractic adjustment
- Reflexology helps the body to heal faster after surgery
- Reflexology reduces pain
- Reflexology improves sleep patterns
- Reflexology sharpens mental alertness
- Reflexology increases the attention span

History of Reflexology

The first findings of Reflexology date back to 2330 B.C., over 5000 years ago. A wall painting was found in the tomb of Ankhmahor (the highest official after the king) at Saqqara near Cairo. One man had his hands on the other man's foot. And the translation read:

"Don't hurt me!" The Egyptian Physician replied, "I shall so you will praise me".

Cleopatra is said to have worked on Mark Anthony's feet in 60 B.C.

Buddha's up-turned foot as a stone carving, with Sanskrit symbols on the sole is found at the Medicine Teacher Temple in Nara, Japan in 700 A.D.

The Incas passed down to the American Indians the use of pressure therapy on the feet. It was taught that it healed the whole body, and it has been passed down through the generations.

It is said that in 1300 A.D., Marco Polo introduced reflex-massage to the west.

Ancient Chinese used pressure points on the feet for healing the whole body.

The first book on Zone therapy was published by two European physicians, Dr. Adamus and Dr. A'tatis in 1582.

The second book on Zone Therapy was published by Dr. Bell in the 19th Century.

In 1870, Russian physician Dr. Ivan Pavlou, founder of the Russian Brain Institute, used Zone therapy.

In 1890, a physician from Germany named Dr. Alfons Cornelius, discovered by trying reflex-massage on certain spots to cure his own disease, that the healing process intensified. He took notes, and in 1898 he published a book called "Druckpunkte," which means "Pressure Points".

In 1913, Zone therapy was brought into America by Dr. William Fitzgerald, a ear, nose, throat surgeon from Connecticut. He used Zone therapy to deaden the pain, and to replace drugs in minor operations. He also used it to relieve the underlying causes. He treated lumps in the breast, uterine fibroids, respiratory problems, and eye conditions. Dr. Fitzgerald was responsible for designing a chart on the longitudinal zones   of the body.
Dr. Bowers a dentist encouraged and helped Dr. Fitzgerald to write his first book called "Relieving Pain at Home," published in 1917.

Dr. Bowers had published a book in the early 1900's called, "Stop that Toothache, Squeeze your Toe". But the medical world did not accept it then.

In 1919, Dr. Joe Riley a D.C. discovered horizontal Zones on the feet and body. He worked with facial and ear points and published a book called "Zone Therapy Simplified". He detailed the first diagrams of the reflex points found on the feet.

In the 1930's, Eunice Ingham, a physiotherapist and a student of Dr. Joe Riley, continued to chart the feet and developed it into Reflexology. In 1938, she published "Stories the Feet Can Tell" and in 1951 she published "Stories the Feet Have Told". After publishing the books she toured America giving workshops.

In 1952 Dr. George Starr White, M.D. traveled the U.S. lecturing doctors the principles of Zone therapy Dr. White states "Zone therapy must be classed with the best and most original procedure in medicine today." Dr. Fitzgerald is to be congratulated upon given to mankind a valuable adjunct in therapy. "The system is simplicity itself, yet the technique must be carried out in an exact manner. It cannot be done in a haphazard way."

In the late 1950's Eunice's niece (Eusebia Messenger, R.N.) and nephew (Dwight Byers) joined her in helping out with the workshops. It grew and they started a school called "National Institute of Reflexology." Since her death in 1974, at the age of 85, Dwight and Eusebia have picked up where Eunice left off.

Dwight Byers renamed the St. Petersburg, FL. school, to "International Institute of Reflexology". Dwight published his book called "Better Health with Reflexology," and he started schools all across the world. If it was not for Dwight , the field of Reflexology would not have gained the acceptance that it has in the past years. Thank you Dwight!!

Possible Reactions During a Reflexology Session

- Expressions of pain - moaning, wincing, pulling away from the practitioner
- Perspiration of the hands and feet, natural way of detoxifying through the skin
- Contraction of muscle groups, especially in the leg area, because of pain
- A feeling of being cold or chilled
- Laughter or smiling through the pain

Possible Reactions After a session
(all positive signs)

- Relaxation or tiredness
- Rejuvenation or more energy
- Feeling of dizziness
- Feeling of nausea
- Frequent urinating; Sometimes the urine is cloudy with an odor, a natural way of detoxifying
- Frequent bowel movements or diarrhea, a natural way of detoxifying
- Emotional releases, such as crying
- Discharge from sinuses or coughing phlegm, a natural way of detoxifying
- A change in sleep patterns, perhaps deeper and calmer
- Rashes or sores, a natural way of detoxifying through the skin

Reflexology Rules for the Practitioner

- Do not diagnose
- Do not treat for a specific condition or illness
- Do not recommend over-the-counter medications, vitamins, or herbs
- Do not adjust medications
- Do not predict future health of the client
- Never use tools on the feet (unless it is for self-help only)

When not to use Reflexology on your Clients

- Trauma to the feet
- Cuts or open sores
- Athlete's foot
- Planters wart
- Varicose veins that are dilated or knotty
- Severe edema
- Ingrown toenail or corn (avoid the area)
- Cracked callous (avoid the area)
- Bruises (avoid the area)
- Pregnancy (especially during first trimester)

Research Studies done on Reflexology

In England the use of Reflexology improved the quality of life for twelve cancer patients.

In Australia, according to a report from the School of Nursing, Division of Science and Design, University of Canberra, ten minute reflexology sessions provided relieve from pain, nausea, and anxiety in cancer patients.

In Greenville, N.C., researchers at the School of Nursing offering help through reflexology for patients suffering from breast and lung cancers found that their patients experienced decrease in anxiety and pain.

The National Board of Health Council, Denmark, in 1995 studied 220 patients with headaches for a three month period. Results showed that 16% said they were cured, 65% said they were helped, and 18% were unchanged.

The FDZ Research Committee, Denmark researched 23 of the worst cases of migraines headaches. After twelve sessions each, the results were 45% no longer had headaches, 30% felt a big improvement, 10% felt a little better, and 15% were unchanged.

Research studies on Type 2 Diabetics at the First Teaching Hospital, Beijing Medical University, this study reported numerous symptoms greatly reduced and that reflexology is an effective therapy for Type 2 Diabetes. For more information on this study log on to the internet at www.pacificreflexology.com/diabetes.htm

The 1996 China Reflexology Symposium Report has found foot reflexology to be 93.63% effective in treating 63 disorders. After analysis of 8,096 clinical cases, Dr. Wang Liang reported reflexology was significantly effective in 48.68% of all the cases, and improved treatment in 44.95% of the cases.

Frequently Asked Questions

How does Reflexology feel during a session?

Very relaxing during and sometimes it comes afterwards. Some of my clients say the feet feel warm and tingling and also in certain areas of the body there some have felt a warming sensation and tingling. Reason is because of better blood and nerve supply. There maybe pain in certain areas, but the pain is a hurt, but feel good pain. It is due to maybe the organ, gland, or part of the body not functioning at its 100%, or it maybe a foot problem. Afterwards most of my clients say that their body feels like every nerve ending has melted !

Can anyone receive Reflexology sessions?

Yes, the only contraindication is pregnant women, some doctors say not in the first trimester and some say not in the last trimester and some say not at all.

Is Reflexology like a massage?

No, in Reflexology you remove only the shoes and socks. The reflexologist uses a thumb-walking technique on specific reflexes of the feet, hand, and sometimes ears, and this relieves stress and reduces pain in the body.

How long does a session last?

Thirty minutes to one hour. If its a child or someone who is very ill, fifteen minutes.

When should I schedule my next appointment?

If it is a chronic problem, every week for one month then watch for the progress, then down to every other week. A diabetic can use it twice weekly, then down to once weekly.

Is Reflexology covered by insurance?

In most states it is not. Just recently in Wisconsin Blue Cross and Blue Shield is covering most alternative therapies including Reflexology. And sometimes if the doctor orders it, then insurance pays a portion.

Can Reflexology cause me any harm?

No, reflexology brings the body back to balance, improves blood, nerve, and oxygen supply. In some cases, reflexology facilitates the body's release of toxins it may cause perspiration, nausea, diarrhea, headache, and cloudiness in the urine. These minor discomforts are our own body's healing process, and the process of elimination helps to carry off toxins.

Can Reflexology be replaced by medical treatments?

No, Reflexology helps to relieve stress and tension. The AMA has stated that "seventy-five percent of illnesses are due to stress." Relieve the stress and tension and the body will go back to a harmonizing balance.

What does "Sensitivity Spots" Mean?

Sensitive spots could mean a foot problem or it could mean an organ, gland, or part of the body is not functioning at 100%, and stress could be the culprit. It is known by the medical profession that 75% of all illnesses are caused by stress.

A client of mine week after week has the same sensitive spots. One week I worked on him right after his vacation and before he had gone back to work. He virtually had no sensitive spots. I realized then, that stress does create havoc in our bodies. After working on several clients I have come to the realization that everybody holds stress in different parts of the body.

Other reason for sensitivity spots are a past surgery. Drugs are another reason for sensitivity spots as they have side effects that causes stress in different parts of the body. Poor nutrition is another reason sensitive spots show up. And you will usually find sensitivity in the digestive system area. Foot problems such as heel spurs, bunion, morton's neuroma, sesamoiditis, and plantar fasciitis also cause sensitivity.

Some people will have sensitive spots on every part of the foot, and some no sensitive spots. For instance, some people have no problem walking over gravel or pebbles and some people creep over the gravel because of sensitivity. The person with sensitive feet has to walk over it and over it before the sensitivity disappears. The same is true with reflexology sessions. Those with sensitive feet will get less and less sensitive with each session.

If a person has no sensitive spots, they could be very healthy, and have very little stress. Or drugs sometimes have a numbing effect.

If you find a sensitive spot, work out the sensitivity. When you find the spot go over it gradually, adding more pressure as you go. Leave it alone for awhile then come back to it, until the pain has diminished. Once I have achieved no sensitivity, I feel I have improved better blood and nerve supply to the areas and relieved the stress from that part of the body.

Can you use Reflexology on Children?

The answer is "Yes," but for a shorter period of time, and use light to moderate pressure. But do not be too gentle, as it may tickle them, and they may not want reflexology treatment because of being tickled.

Many of my clients ask, "At what age can you start working on children?" You can start using reflexology as early as infancy. In my experiences, reflexology helps with colicky babies and constipation.

I have had great luck using Reflexology on children for ADD and AD/HD, bed-wetting, and constipation. The children seem to be very receptive to the treatment. They look at me very intently as I am working on them. Most children seem happy to having their feet worked on. I have run into parents and grandparents of children whom I have worked on and they tell me that the children ask to have more reflexology sessions.

Steps in working children's feet:

1. use relaxing techniques (make it fun for them)

2. use light pressure (not too light, avoid tickling them)

3. keep your eye on the child for any tenderness

4. communicate with the child.

Reflexology on Children with A.D.D. and A.D./H.D.

I have had great results using reflexology on children with ADD and AD/HD in just 10 minute sessions a day.

ADD is a disorder that children are diagnosed with when they are having difficulty paying attention, not listening or following directions. The problem seems to stem from an area in the brain involving frontal lobe and basil ganglia which is under-active.

AD/HD is a neurobiological disorder attributed to a deficiency of dopamine. Children display such problems as impulsive behavior, short attention span, fidgeting, squirming in their chair, getting up from class to walk or run around, talking impulsively, and speaking before thinking.

I wanted to help parents search for an alternative to help their child with ADD and AD/HD without the use of medication. I am concerned that too many children are prescribed Ritalin for attention deficit disorder and hyperactivity. It is a stimulant that speeds up the brain so fast that the brain shifts into neutral.

I am familiar with a child that was diagnosed with AD/HD and was not on medication. I watched this child hitting his friend and acting hyper and talking loudly. I suggested, "Come here, take your shoes off, and put your feet on my lap". He said "Okay." I started on his right foot and found the sensitive spots were adrenal and hypothalamus. After working on those sensitive spots, there was a BIG sigh of relief. The sensitivity spots were the same on the left foot, and once again another BIG sigh. The child actually rolled his eyes in the back of his head as he was very relaxed after the session. He hugged me and thanked me and I could tell all the anxiety had disappeared. He walked me out to my car when I was ready to go. I noticed he walked very slowly, and I could tell he was ready to go to sleep!

Why was the adrenal reflex area sensitive? The adrenal is the inner gland that secretes the hormone adrenaline. By pressing on the adrenal reflex on the foot it helps to secrete adrenaline in the body to help with physical and emotional stress.

Why was the hypothalamus reflex area sensitive? The hypothalamus is located in the brain and the role that it plays is the expression of emotions. By pressing on the hypothalamus reflex, several hormones are released, one of which is dopamine, and that is what these children with AD/HD are deficient of - dopamine. This hormone is released into the bloodstream and travels to the anterior lobe of the pituitary.

In chapter 7, look up ADD and AD/HD in the endocrine disorders to learn how to work the reflex areas.

Can I use Reflexology on the Elderly?

Reflexology is very beneficial for the elderly because they often do not get physically touched. Most of the time they do not get enough exercise. Reflexology improves better blood and oxygen supply to every organ, gland, and part of the body. Reflexology helps with stiffness and pain due to arthritis.

Dr. Jesus Manzanares a medical doctor, surgeon, and is the Secretary of Health Services in Catalonia. He began his investigations in Reflexology because his grandmother had rheumatism and was treated by conventional means without results. His grandmother heard of reflexology and tried it and got results!

Steps on working on the elderly:

- work lightly to begin with then gradually work up to moderate pressure

- shorter amount of time 30 minutes is sufficient.

Can you use Reflexology on Cancer Patients?

In the past few years there has been interest in the field of Complementary and Alternative therapies for treatments of cancer. Many years ago it was thought that massage therapy and reflexology would spread the cancer around in the body. Recently there has been research on alternative therapies at the teaching hospitals across the world. No cures have been documented, but research found that Reflexology did reduce stress, tension, and anxiety. Therefore, Reflexology assisted other medical treatment to put the cancer patient into remission.

Once you find that you may have cancer, emotional stress comes in to play and may cause nervousness and anxiety. The brain then signals the adrenal glands to produce a chemical, corticosteroid, that weakens the immune system.

Researchers in the field of psychoneuroimmunology have documented links between emotion and biochemical events of the body, therefore establishing on a scientific basis what folk healers have always known: emotions can manifest themselves as physical symptoms. A women's health expert, Christiane Northrup, M.D. of Maine, believes that emotions help to generate symptoms that keep illnesses in place. She believes that emotions are legitimate toxins, contributing to weakening the immune system.

Reflexology helps the body to relax and to reduce anxiety. Reflexology could cause cancer to go into remission. Reflexology also could strengthen the immune system. If surgery is performed, reflexology helps to improve better blood supply, nerve supply, and oxygen to speed up the healing process.

1. Use the relaxing techniques.

2. Use light to moderate pressure.

3. Work only a maximum of 30 minutes.

4. Work all the reflexes in the feet to give better blood and nerve supply to every organ, gland, and part of the body. All systems support each other.

5. Do not miss the hypothalamus as it has a role in the expressions of emotions: such as, fear and pain.

6. Do not miss the adrenal gland as it affects the immune system.

In my experiences in working with terminally ill cancer patients, after a session they feel relaxed and also invigorated. In the case of one of my clients who had bone, brain, liver, and lung cancer, the doctors could virtually do nothing more for him. After the Reflexology session he paced the floor saying "I feel like I'm 16 again, I feel so good !!"

With my clients who are undergoing chemotherapy, the response after a session is that they feel the nausea disappear and have more energy.

* **Before embarking on any alternative program make sure you talk to your physician.**

Can I use Reflexology on Pregnant women? Reflexology in the Birthing Rooms

There are contraindications of using reflexology throughout the pregnancy, avoid working the reproductive organs. It may cause contractions. In an other hand many other reflexologist have safely worked on many pregnant women, but they say to avoid doing reflexology during the first trimester.

Dr. Gowri Motha an obstetrician and reflexologist is the pioneer of water births in London, she reports that certain maternity conditions may contraindicate reflexology.

Dr. Jesus Manzanares a medical doctor and surgeon, he reports, not to work the reproductive organs on pregnant women throughout the pregnancy because it may cause contractions.

Nurses and midwives are using reflexology at the National Maternity Hospital in Dublin, Ireland, they began in 1995 because of doctors and patients and midwives insisting on the reflexology treatment because they found the results to be positive and the benefits enormous. It is reported that labor can be induced, it increases the strength of the contractions, to calm down contractions if they are in extreme pain, help with expelling the placenta, helping with urinary retention after delivery, post-natal depression, and PMS.

In the book called "Zone Therapy" written by three medical doctors in 1917, in chapter 6 they write about "painless childbirth". Dr. Nesbitt, of Waukegan, IL. is one of a number of physicians who have had practical experience with zone therapy during childbirth, he reports that when strong contractions began, he pressed on the dorsal part of the each foot and it relieved the pain, he exerted pressure for about three minutes at a time, and his patients had no pain what so ever. Another point is that after the babies were born the women did not experience fatigue and the babies were more active than usual.

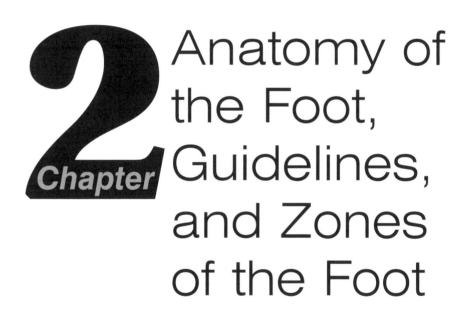

2 Chapter Anatomy of the Foot, Guidelines, and Zones of the Foot

Bones of the Foot

There are 26 bones in the foot

- **Phalanges-** are the bones of the toes. There are two bones for the great toe- the proximal and distal. The other toes have three bones- the distal, middle,and the proximal. They connect to the metatarsal heads.

- **Metatarsal-** there are five metatarsal bones across the foot. The head of the first metatarsal is two sesamoid bones on the plantar surface. The first, second and third metatarsal connect to the first, second and third cuneiforms. And the fourth and fifth metatarsal connect to the cuboid.

- **Sesamoid bones-** are rounded bones embedded in some of the tendons. They are connected the the first metatarsal head.

- **Cuneiforms-** there are three cuneiforms. They are connected to three metatarsals, the navicular and cuboid.

- **Navicular-** sits on the medial side of the foot. It connects to the talus, and the three cuneiforms.

- **Cuboid-** sits on the lateral side of the foot. It is connected to the fourth and fifth metatarsals, and to the lateral cuneiform, and then to the calcaneus.

- **Calcaneus-** is the largest bone in the foot and it forms the heel. It is connected to the talus and to the anterior side of the cuboid.

- **Talus-** is the upper part of the foot bone; it forms the ankle joint. It is connected to the tibia and the fibula on the upper surface.

- **On the next page is the diagram of the bones of the foot.**

Bones of the Foot

Medial View

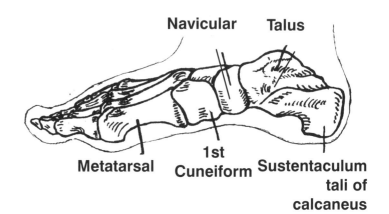

Navicular   Talus

Metatarsal   1st Cuneiform   Sustentaculum tali of calcaneus

Plantar View

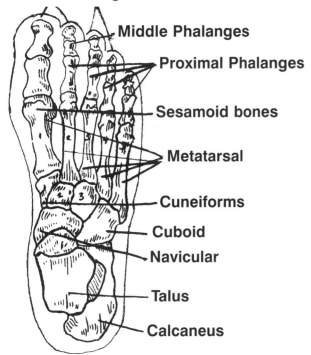

Distal Phalanges

Middle Phalanges

Proximal Phalanges

Sesamoid bones

Metatarsal

Cuneiforms

Cuboid

Navicular

Talus

Calcaneus

Lateral View

Talus   Navicular

Cuneiforms

Calcaneus   Cuboid   Metatarsal

Front View of the Foot Muscles

There are twelve tendons at the end of the muscles that attach the muscles to bone. There are also one hundred-seven ligaments they hold bones together and helps with movement.

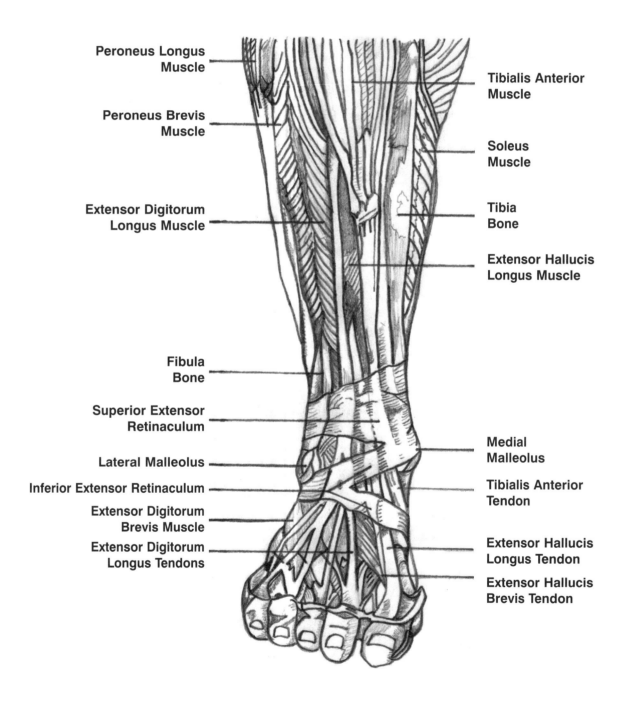

Back View of the Foot Muscles

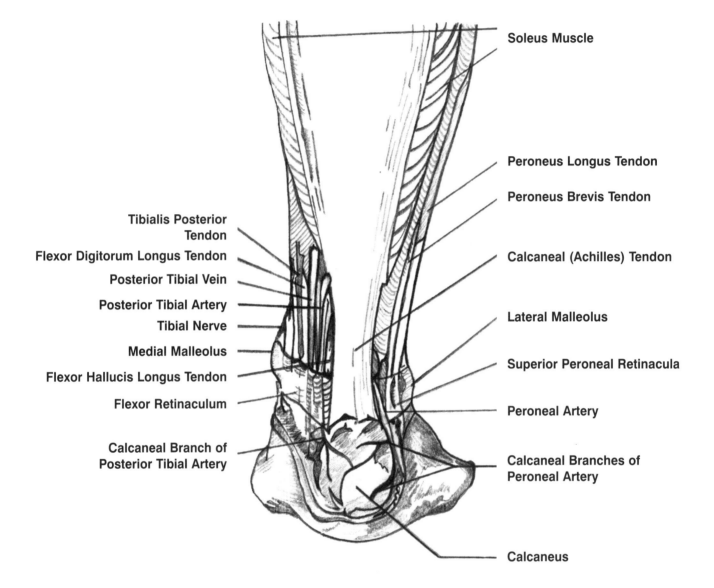

Soleus Muscle

Peroneus Longus Tendon

Peroneus Brevis Tendon

Calcaneal (Achilles) Tendon

Lateral Malleolus

Superior Peroneal Retinacula

Peroneal Artery

Calcaneal Branches of
Peroneal Artery

Calcaneus

Tibialis Posterior
Tendon

Flexor Digitorum Longus Tendon

Posterior Tibial Vein

Posterior Tibial Artery

Tibial Nerve

Medial Malleolus

Flexor Hallucis Longus Tendon

Flexor Retinaculum

Calcaneal Branch of
Posterior Tibial Artery

Side View of the Foot Muscles and Tendons

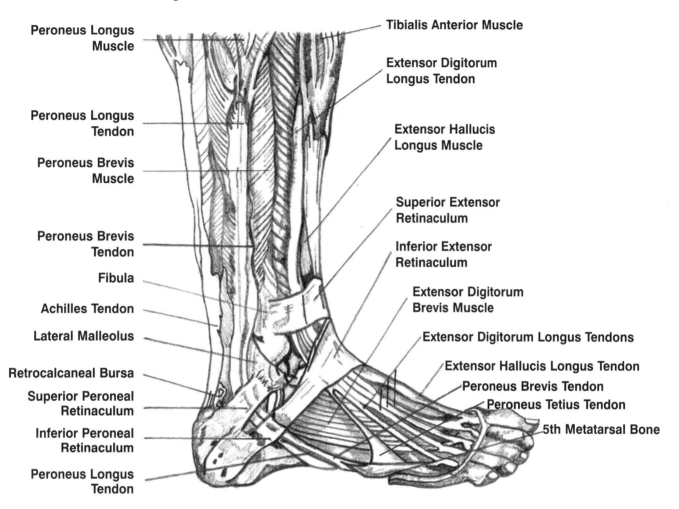

Peroneus Longus
Muscle

Peroneus Longus
Tendon

Peroneus Brevis
Muscle

Peroneus Brevis
Tendon

Fibula

Achilles Tendon

Lateral Malleolus

Retrocalcaneal Bursa

Superior Peroneal
Retinaculum

Inferior Peroneal
Retinaculum

Peroneus Longus
Tendon

Tibialis Anterior Muscle

Extensor Digitorum
Longus Tendon

Extensor Hallucis
Longus Muscle

Superior Extensor
Retinaculum

Inferior Extensor
Retinaculum

Extensor Digitorum
Brevis Muscle

Extensor Digitorum Longus Tendons

Extensor Hallucis Longus Tendon

Peroneus Brevis Tendon

Peroneus Tetius Tendon

5th Metatarsal Bone

View of the Plantar Muscles

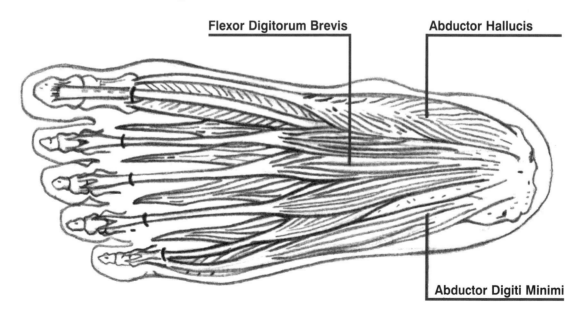

Flexor Digitorum Brevis

Abductor Hallucis

Abductor Digiti Minimi

Terms of
Anatomical Direction

Anterior -   towards the front of the body, or in front of.

Posterior -   towards the back of the body, or behind.

Distal-   the farthest away from the center part of the body.

Proximal-   the closest to the center of the body.

Lateral-   the outside of the body or the outside of the foot.

Medial-   the closest to the center of the body or inside of the foot.

Dorsal-   top part of the foot or hand.

Palmar-   the bottom of the hand.

Plantar-   the bottom of the foot.

Deep-   below the surface.

Superficial-   on top of the surface.

Plantar flexion-   the foot bending downward.

Terms of Anatomical Direction

Dorsiflexion- the foot bending upward.

Abduction- the foot moving away from the mid-line of the body.

Adduction- the foot moving towards the mid-line of the body.

Pronation- three plane movement: abduction, eversion, and dorsiflexion.

Supination- three plane movement: adduction, inversion, and plantar flexion.

Inversion- the plantar part of the foot turning inward toward the mid-line of the body.

Eversion- the plantar part of the foot turning outward away from the mid-line of the body.

Pulse of the Foot

The location of the Doralis pedis pulse is on the top and center of the foot in line with the 2nd toe.

The location of the Post Tibial pulse is on the inside of the foot between the ankle and achilles tendon.

Move your finger slowly until you find the pulse.

Biomechanics

Biomechanics is the study of the mechanical laws of human motion, purposefully movements of the lower leg and foot.

The motions of a ballet dancer, or a runner in full, are examples of perfect biomechanics in action. Podiatrist and researchers are seeking to understand abnormal walking and running motions. This was inspired because of the running/jogging phase and the problems that came with it. They are understanding why normal and abnormal weight bearing has been shown to affect parts of the body from the lower back to the ankle. The overuse of the runners/joggers with biomechanical faults has proven to be the culprit of lower limb and back problems, over seventy-five percent of complaints are related to poor mechanical function of the lower leg and foot.

The walking/gait cycle is the person's range of motion when they are moving forward. This cycle is divided into two phases: stance and swing. The biomechanics of the weight-bearing foot during these phases is to see if the person is walking or running normally.

The stance phase of the gait cycle is divided into three separate stages: contact begins at the heel-strike, the second stage is mid-stance is when the front part of the foot makes contact with the ground, the final stage of the stance phase is called propulsive it starts at heel-lift and ends at toe-off that is when the foot totally leaves the ground and does not bear weight. The parts of the stance account for two-thirds of the total weight.

The other third of the total weight of the gait cycle is the swing phase. It is not divided into different mechanisms because it occurs when the foot is totally off the ground and not bearing any weight.

The basic fault occurs when an abnormal amount of weight is bearing on a specific part of the foot; and the cause of the abnormal weight-bearing process are biomechanical an abnormal pronation and supination. This can lead to foot problems. When you allow a biomechanical fault to continue you are helping along the wear-and- tear process in the joints in your feet, legs, hips, and lower back, this is constantly stressing the joints in order to walk or run.

Pronation involves three biomechanical movements of the foot during the stance phase: abduction (the foot moving away from the mid-line of the body), eversion (the plantar part of the foot turning outward away from the mid-line of the body), dorsiflexion (the foot bending upward).

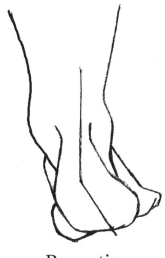

Pronation

Supination is opposite of pronation it involves three opposite biomechanical movements: inversion (the plantar part of the foot turning inward toward the mid-line of the body), adduction (the foot moving towards the mid-line of the body), plantar flexion (the foot bending downward). Supination happens during the last part of the stance phase, from the beginning of the propulsive stage to when the foot lifts off the ground.

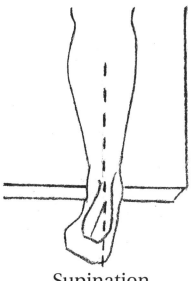

Supination

Abnormal pronation is the major cause of foot problems, occurs when the foot pronates when it should be supinating, or it over-pronates during a normal pronation period of the gait cycle. A foot supinates when it should be pronating, or when exceeds a normal amount of supination. These five bony abnormalities are found to create abnormal pronation: forefoot valgus (plantar-flexed first metatarsal bone), a plantar-flexed fifth metatarsal head, forefoot valgus deformity, a rear foot varus deformity, and a lack of motion in the ankle joint.

Abnormal supination accounts for a small percentage of all foot problems. The supinating foot is one with a high arch and rigid structure, or a neuro-muscular component to the problem causing the supination syndrome.

Abduction is when the foot moves laterally away from the mid-line of the body.

Adduction is when the foot moves medially moving towards the mid-line of the body.

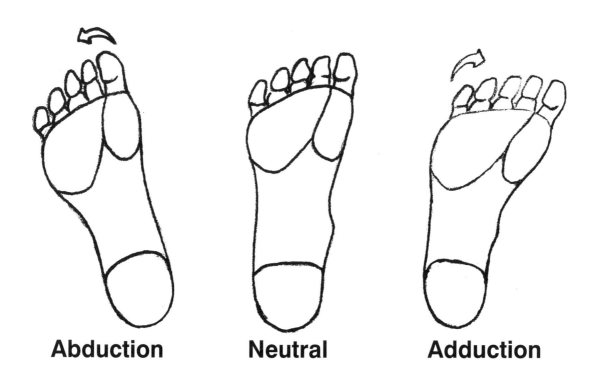

Abduction   **Neutral**   **Adduction**

Eversion is when the foot twists outward and upward away from the mid-line of the body.

Inversion is when the foot twists inward and upward towards the mid-line of the body.

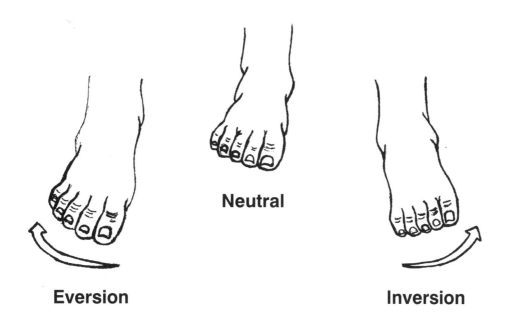

Neutral

Eversion   **Inversion**

Dorsiflexion is when the foot bends upwards towards the tibia.

Plantar flexion is when the foot plantar bends downward away from the tibia.

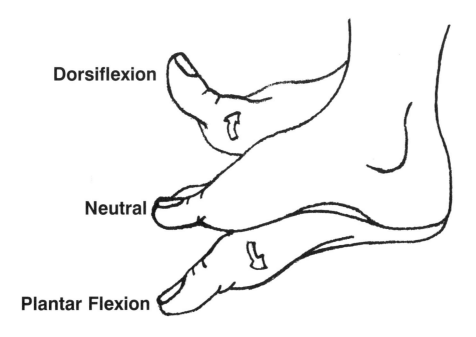

Dorsiflexion

Neutral

Plantar Flexion

Guidelines to the Feet

Remember that from the tips of the toes to the baseline of the toes on both feet, are all brain and neck reflexes.

From the baseline of the toes to the diaphragm line on both feet is the heart, respiratory, thymus, breast, chest, spine, and shoulder reflexes.

From the diaphragm line to the waistline on the right foot is the liver/gallbladder, adrenal, duodenum, kidney, head of the pancreas, and solar plexus. On the left foot it is the adrenal, stomach, spleen, spine, solar plexus, kidney, and pancreas.

From the waistline to the heel line on the right foot is the ileocecal valve, ascending colon, transverse colon, small intestines, ureter tube, and bladder. On the left foot is the transverse colon, descending colon, small intestines, spine, ureter tube, and bladder.

Below the heel line on the right foot is the sciatic nerve, rectum, hip/knee/leg, and spine. The left foot is the same.

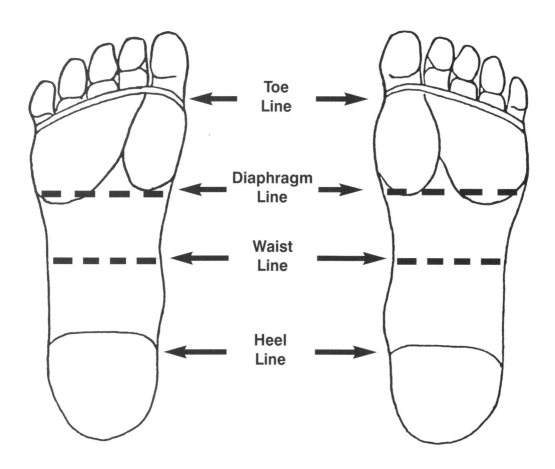

Learn to Locate the Zones in the Body and the Feet

The Zone Theory and Zone Chart was developed by Dr. Fitzgerald. He believed that there are ten invisible electrical currents that run lengthwise through the body from head to toe. With five zones on the right side of the body, and five zones on the left, our whole organism is divided into ten zones they are in line with the toes and fingers. By applying pressure with the thumbs at the bottom of the foot in a zone, it will affect the entire zone throughout the body. The pressure releases energy to unblock any nerve blockage, and aids better blood supply in that zone.

Using the zone chart on the next page, imagine ten zones, starting from the great toe as Zone one. With each toe representing a zone, draw an imaginary line starting from the toe up the leg, through the body and ending at the head. You can take any internal organ in the body and decide what zone line it passes through according to this chart. Then picture in your mind on what part of the foot this line would be found and this will guide you in finding the reflex area.

The 10 Body Zones Mapped on the Feet

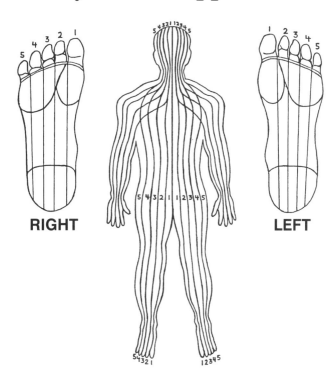

RIGHT   LEFT

The Meridian Theory

The meridian theory states that the human body has fourteen invisible meridians (six yin and six yang) they carry energy throughout the body linking to every organ, gland, and part of the body. The body contains five pairs of vital organs, each of which nourish the body and perform all the functions of sustaining life. These vital organs are the lung-large intestines; stomach-spleen and pancreas; heart-small intestines; bladder-kidneys; gallbladder-liver. In meridian theory chi (energy) runs from one meridian to the next in a continuous circuit, so the lung meridian ends close to the large intestines meridian starts; where the large intestines finishes the stomach meridian starts and etc. The connections between the meridians provide an even amount of circulation of chi, creating a balance of yin and yang.

In addition to the five pairs of vital organs meridians, there are four other major meridians - called the heart protector and triple heater; the governing and conception vessels. Yin and yang meridians are two channels that traverse the mid-line of the body. The yin meridians are in the front and inside body surfaces; the yang meridians are in the back and outside body surfaces.

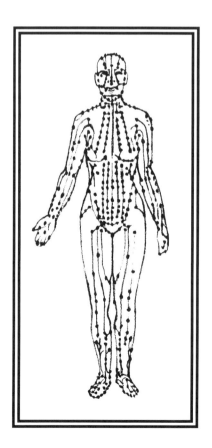

Referral Areas

If a limb is injured, such as the foot, you will have to work the referral area, which would be the hand on the same side of the body. Work on the hand in the same zone as the injury is located on the foot, as they correspond to each other.

Here are the areas of referral to different areas of the body.

If this part of the body is injured, then work the:

Foot ....Hand

Hand ....Foot

Plantar part of the foot ....Palmar of the hand

Dorsal part of the foot......................................Top of the hand

Great toe ....Thumb

Small toes ....Fingers

Ankle..Wrist

Calf ....Forearm

Knee ....Elbow

Thigh ....Upper Arm

Hip ....Shoulder

Quiz on Anatomy of the Foot, Guidelines, and the Zones

1. How many bones are in each foot?
   A) 24   B) 21   C) 26

2. How many tendons on each foot?
   A) 12   B) 16   C) 7

3. How many ligaments on each foot?
   A) 100   B) 112   C) 107

4. What part of the foot is medial?
   A) inside   B) outside   C) top

5. What anatomical direction is plantar flexion?
   A) foot bending upward
   B) foot moving away from mid-line of the body
   C) foot bending downwards

6. What part of the body does the baseline of the toes represent?
   A) lung and heart   B) head and neck   C) colon areas

7. How many zones in the body and feet?
   A) 12   B) 10   C) 5

8. Where is the fifth zone located?
   A) lateral side   B) medial side

9. If the foot was injured what referral area would you work?
   A) thumb   B) hand   C) dorsal side

10. If the elbow was injure what referral area would you work?
    A) hip   B) ankle   C) knee

*Answer key on page 325

3 Chapter

Holding and Thumb & Finger-Walking Techniques

Basic Holding, Thumb-Walking, and Finger-Walking Techniques

Thumb-walking is used on most reflex areas. You take the tip of the thumb and bend the thumb at the first joint so the thumb can do the little steps in caterpillar walking. Avoid bending any other joint . Practice these small caterpillar steps on your hand or forearm, as your thumb bends at the first joint it moves your thumb forward. This thumb-walking movement is always going forward, not sideways or backwards. Keep practicing making sure these caterpillar steps are small steps because you need to make them small enough to work the 7,200 nerve endings that exist at the bottom of the feet.

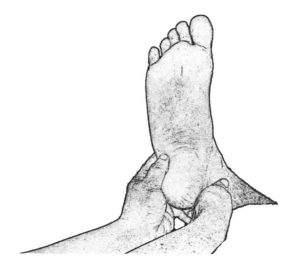

Finger-walking is the same as thumb-walking. Use the tip of the index finger and bend only the first joint and use the small caterpillar steps to practice on your forearm or hand. Use finger-walking while working the breast/chest reflex areas of the feet.

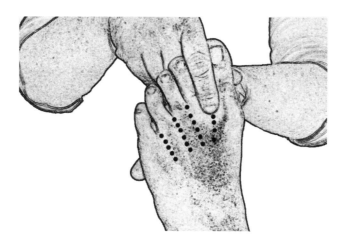

Finger-rocking is used only while working the brain reflex areas. You rock your index finger back and forth at the tip of each toe.

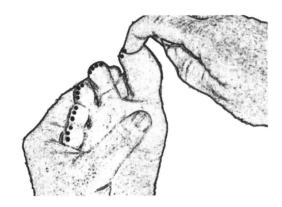

Hook-back and release is used for working the pituitary, hypothalamus, and pineal glands. Upon finding the reflex area hook in with the thumb and pull the thumb backwards, then release.

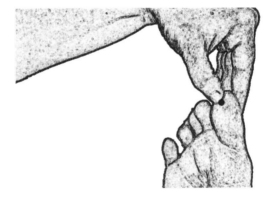

Thumb-press is pressing the thumb into a reflex point. When the thumb-press is required, press on a count of nine, release and repeat.

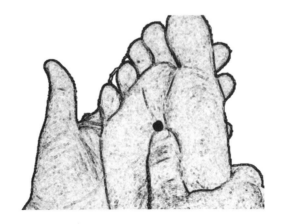

The amount of pressure that you will be using will be light at the beginning until you have mastered the art of the thumb and finger- walking technique, make sure you use and even amount of pressure with every little walking step that you do. When you have mastered the walking step start practicing on getting deeper with every walking step. Use approximately two to ten pounds of pressure. Note: always keep you eye on the client if it is too much pain for them back off and work another reflex area and the come back to the tender reflex and work it out.

The Reflexology process: have your client sit with legs raised in a reclining position preferably in a Lafuma free gravity chair. Powder or very little lotion maybe used to allow greater ease of hand movement. To buy the chair look to the internet and go into your favorite search engine and type Lafuma free gravity chair. Also gardening stores may have the chairs and RV and camping stores.

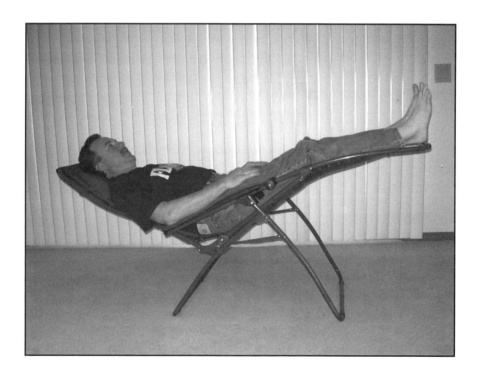

4 Chapter Relaxing Techniques

Foot Stimulating

Place the palms of your hands on each side of the foot at the metatarsal region. This is a fast inversion and eversion of the foot. Lightly slap the dorsal (top) of the foot.

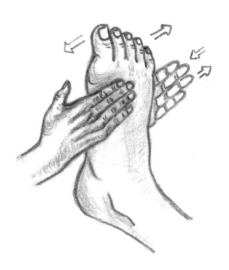

Foot Stimulating

Place the heels of your hands firmly on each side of the talus (ankle). Move the heels of your hands back and forth (do not rub the skin). This is a fast inversion and eversion of the ankle and foot.

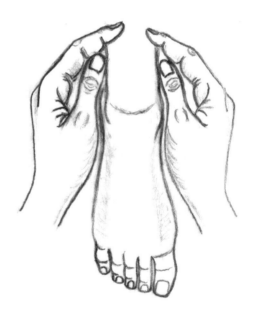

Diaphragm Relax

With your holding hand, gently pull up on all toes. Place your thumb on the diaphragm line and with holding hand gently pull the foot over the thumb. Work across the diaphragm line.

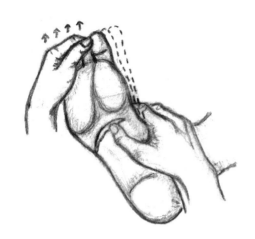

Ankle Circling

With the holding hand, rest the heel of the foot on the palm of the hand. Grasp the medial (inside) part of the foot near the toes and with the working hand make a circle with the foot. Then reverse the circle.

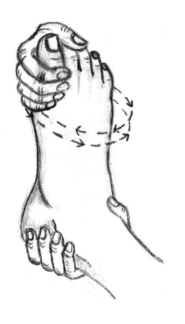

Toe Circling

With your holding hand, firmly hold the metatarsal part of the foot. With your working hand gently pull up on the toe with your thumb and fingers to make a circle.

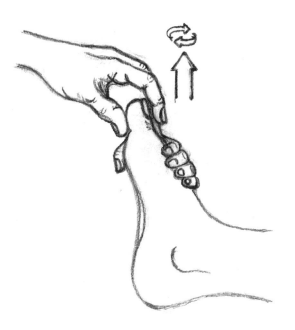

Spinal Twisting

Using both hands, firmly place them together on the medial (inside) part of the foot. The hand closest to the talus (ankle) stays stationary and the other hand gently twists. Both hands slowly work up towards the toes.

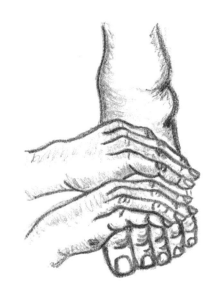

Chapter 5

Central Nervous System

The Central Nervous System

The Central Nervous System is divided into two parts: the brain and the spinal cord both containing nerve fibers. The peripheral nervous system, which is all the nerves that radiate from the spinal cord, and the solar plexus are the network of nerves throughout your body. This system controls communication from the brain to all parts of the body and from all parts of the body back to the brain.

The Brain is the receiver and the analyzer of the sensory information. It weighs approximately three pounds. It contains neurons (nerve cells). It has three main regions:

1. **The Forebrain:** it contains 70% neurons (nerve cells).

   • **Cerebrum:** is located on the upper part of the forebrain. It is divided into two hemispheres which look like each other, but not in function. It controls perception of senses, origin of body movements, and influences mood and strong emotions such as fear and rage.

   • **Hypothalamus:** is located at the base of the forebrain below the Thalamus. It controls body temperature, blood pressure, sleep, emotions, thirst, appetite, urine release, movement of food through the digestive tract, and controls heart rate. It is the source of eight hormones, two of which pass through the pituitary.

   • **Thalamus:** is located deep in the forebrain. Information from all sensory receptors except smell is processed in the Thalamus before being sent to the cerebral cortex.

2. **The Midbrain:** is the passage of forebrain and hindbrain.

3. **The Hindbrain:**

   • **Cerebellum:** is located at the rear of the brain stem. It controls coordination of muscle groups, equilibrium and balance.

• **Medulla Oblongata:** is located above the spinal cord and below the pons, looking like a swollen tip to the spinal cord. Nerve impulses originate here. It controls breathing and regulates the heartbeat. It is the cross over point from spinal cord to brain.

• **Pons:** is located in the front of the cerebellum, between the medulla and the midbrain. It contains a bundle of fibers that connect to the muscles of the body via the spinal cord to the cerebellum. The Pons contains neurons that control states of arousal while awake. It carries signals from the cerebral cortex to the cerebellum. Nerve impulses from the sense organs are sent to the cerebellum. The Pons helps in the regulation of breathing.

The **Brain reflexes** are located at the tip of each great toe, and fine tuning for the brain is at the tip of each phalanges (toes). Use your index finger and rock at the tip of the toe side to side. The brain is made up of two hemispheres; the left controls the right side of the body, and right controls the left side of the body.

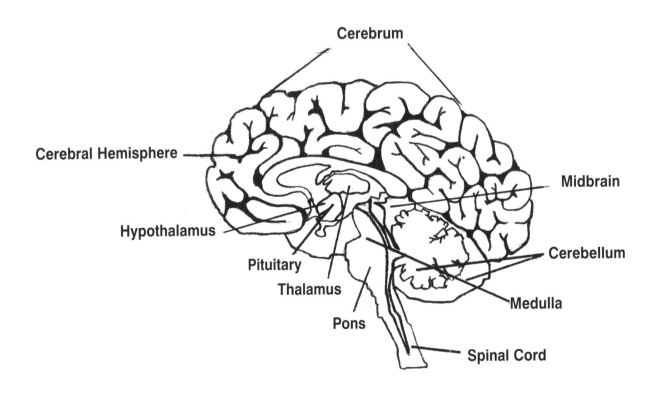

The Spinal Cord is a long hollow tube of neurons (nerve cells) traveling to and from the brain. This hollow tube contains cerebro-spinal fluid. The spinal cord is the communication link between the brain and the peripheral nervous system. The spinal cord consists of 8 cervical, 12 thoracic, 5 lumbar, 5 sacral, and 1 coccyx bone. There are 31 pairs of spinal nerves (peripheral) that exit the spinal cord. These nerves connect to every organ, gland and area of the body.

Cervical 1-8 neck region. The reflex areas for this region are on both feet on the medial (inside) part of the great toe. The 7th and 8th cervical starts at the medial (inside) baseline of the great toe and the 1st cervical is almost to the tip of the great toe. Thumb-walk or finger-walk this area.

Thoracic 1-12 mid-back region. The reflex areas are on the medial (inside) part of both feet. The 1st thoracic starts almost at the baseline of the great toe and the 12th ends a little past the waistline. Thumb-walk this area.

Lumbar 1-5 low back region. The reflex areas are on the medial (inside) part of both feet. The 1st lumbar starts one inch past the waistline and the 5th at the heel line. Thumb-walk this area.

Sacrum and Coccyx tailbone region. The reflex areas are on the medial side of both feet. The sacral and coccyx starts one inch below the heel line and ends at the heel line.

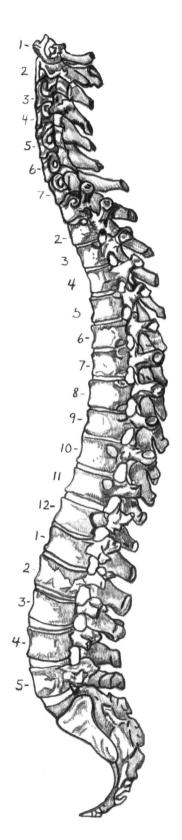

The Nervous System also includes the peripheral nerves, which run from the spinal cord to all organs, glands, and all parts of the body. By stimulating the spinal reflexes you can be promoting better blood and nerve supply to these areas.

Vertebrae	Areas that it corresponds to:
1C	Blood supply to the head, pituitary, scalp, bones of the face, brain, middle and inner ear
2C	Eyes, optic nerves, auditory nerves, sinuses, mastoid bones, tongue
3C	Cheeks, outer ear, teeth, trifacial nerves
4C	Nose, lips, mouth, eustachian tube
5C	Vocal cords, neck glands, pharynx
6C	Neck muscles, shoulders, tonsils
7C	Thyroid gland, shoulder, arm, elbow
1T	Forearm, wrist, hand, fingers, esophagus, trachea
2T	Heart
3T	Lungs, bronchial tubes, breast, chest
4T	Gallbladder

Vertebrae	Areas that it corresponds to:
5T	Liver, solar plexus
6T	Stomach
7T	Duodenum, pancreas
8T	Diaphragm, spleen
9T	Adrenal
10T	Kidneys
11T	Kidneys, ureter tubes
12T	Small colon, lymph gland
1L	Large colon
2L	Appendix, ileocecal valve
3L	Reproductive organs, bladder, knees
4L	Prostate gland, muscles of the lower back, sciatic nerve
5L	Lower legs, ankles, feet
Sacral	Hip, buttocks
Coccyx	Rectum, anus

The Sciatic Nerve is the longest nerve in both legs. The sciatic begins in the lumbar region in the low back and extends through the buttock area to send nerve impulses down to the lower limbs.

Pain from an irritated sciatic nerve is called "sciatica." The pain is felt at the back of the thigh. Sciatica is usually a herniated disc pressing on the nerve.

The reflex areas are located on both plantar part of the calcaneus (heel) half way from the heel line and back of the heel. Thumb-walk this area across from medial to lateral. *Note: this area is often calloused; you may need firmer pressure.

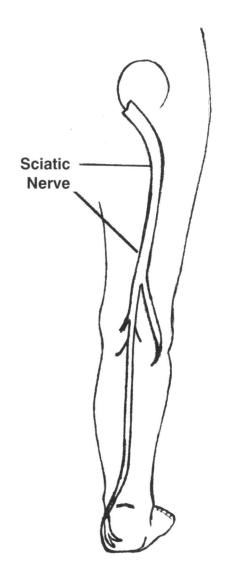

Sciatic
Nerve

Solar Plexus is a network of nerves in the center of the body. It is located behind the stomach. It is part of the autonomic system. This system controls the internal organs.

The reflex areas are on both feet, plantar(bottom) part, in the middle of the diaphragm line. Thumb-press this area.

Locate the Reflex Areas of the Central Nervous System

*Use colored pencils and draw in the reflex areas

A) Brain

B) Solar Plexus

C) 1-7 Cervical

D) 1-12 Thoracic

E) 1-5 Lumbar

F) Sacral

G) Coccyx

H) Sciatic Nerve

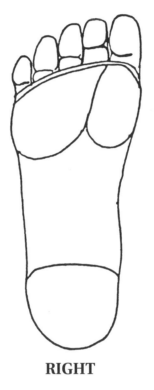

RIGHT

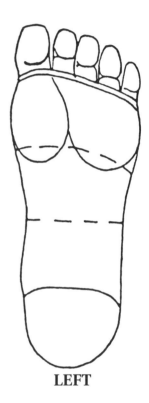

LEFT

*Answer key on next page

Answer Key for Central Nervous System

Brain

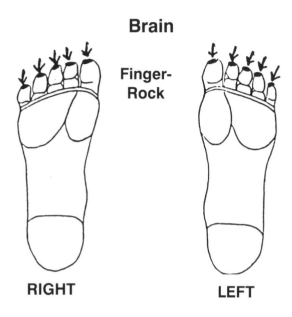

Finger-
Rock

RIGHT　　　　LEFT

Solar Plexus

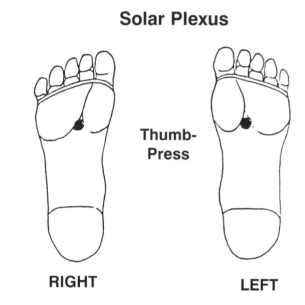

Thumb-
Press

RIGHT　　　　LEFT

1-7 Cervical

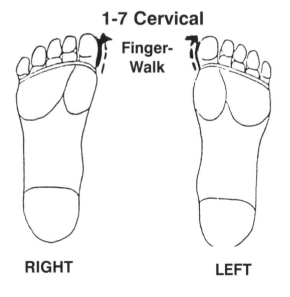

Finger-
Walk

RIGHT　　　　LEFT

1-12 Thoracic

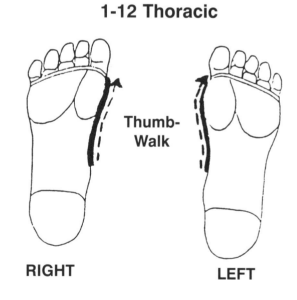

Thumb-
Walk

RIGHT　　　　LEFT

Answer Key for Central Nervous System

1-5 Lumbar

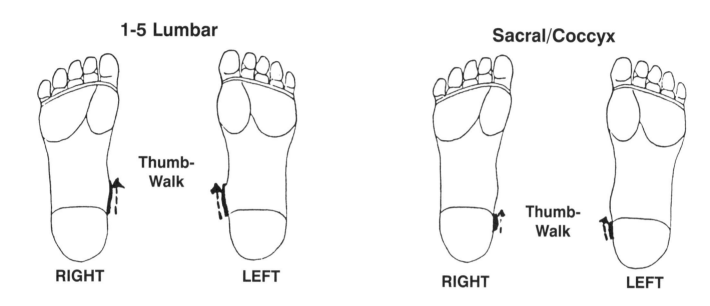

Sacral/Coccyx

Sciatic Nerve

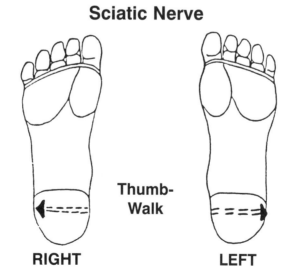

How to Work the
Central Nervous System Reflex Areas

The **Brain reflex areas** are on the tips of both great toes and brain fine-tuning is on tip of all small toes. Finger-rock these areas.

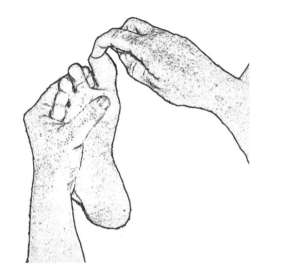
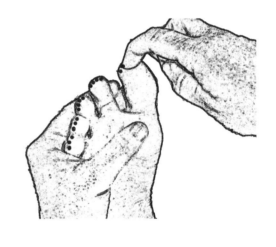

The **Solar Plexus reflex areas** are on both feet under the diaphragm line in zones 2 - 3. Thumb-press this area.

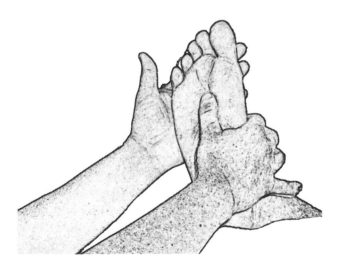
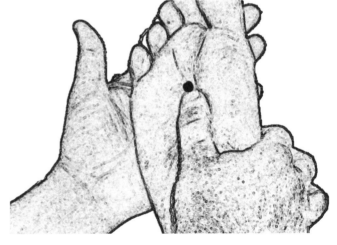

The **Sacral and Coccyx spinal reflex areas** are on both feet on the medial (inside) part in Zone 1; they start just one inch below the heel line and ends at the heel line. Thumb-walk this area.

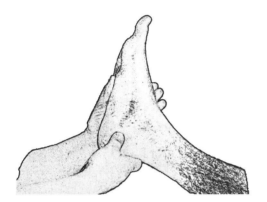 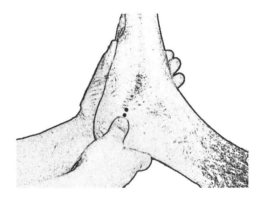

The **Lumbar spinal reflex areas** are on both feet on the medial (inside) part in Zone 1; they start just above the heel line and end two inches above the heel line. Thumb-walk this area.

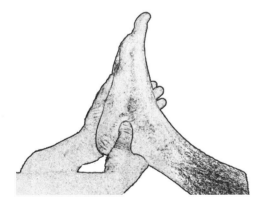 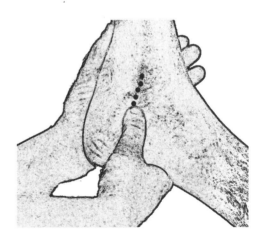

The **Thoracic spinal reflex areas** are on both feet on the medial (inside) part in Zone 1; they start just two inches from the heel line and go to the baseline of the great toe. Thumb-walk this area.

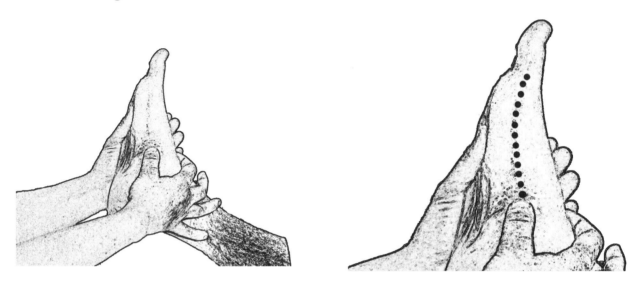

The **Cervical spinal reflex areas** are on both feet on the medial (inside) part in Zone 1; they start from the base of the great toe to one quarter inch from the tip of the toe. Thumb-walk this area.

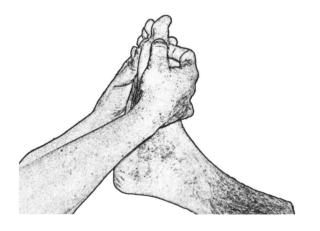
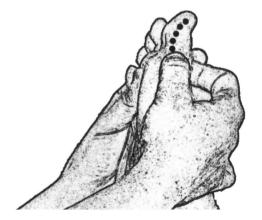

The **Sciatic Nerve reflex areas** are on both feet on the plantar (bottom) calcaneous (heel). Thumb-walk across this area.

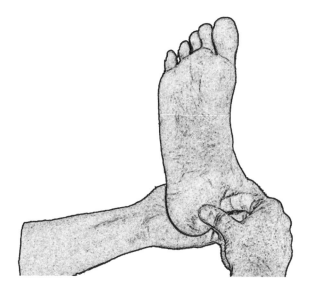 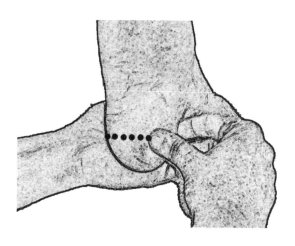

Central Nervous Disorders and the Helper Reflexes

Bells Palsy is a paralyzed facial muscle and the muscle becomes weakened.

Direct reflex- Brain (great toe)

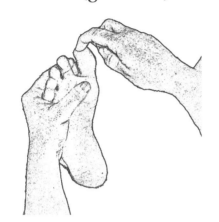 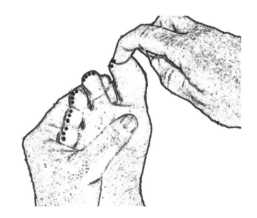

Helper Reflexes- All neck reflexes for better blood supply and cervical for the peripheral nerve that leads to the face.

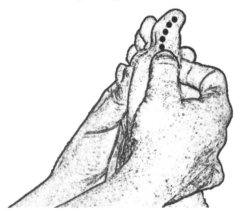 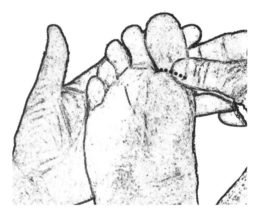

Solar Plexus to relax tension.

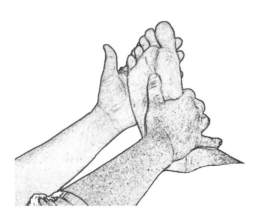 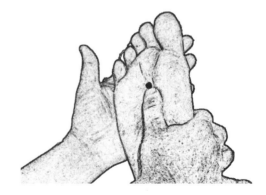

A headache is merely a symptom of another problem in the body. They could be brought on by eye strain, sinus problems, hormone imbalances, neck problems, and tension.

Direct reflex- Brain (great toe)

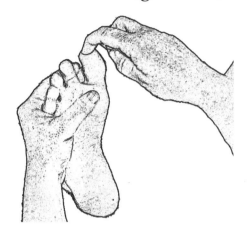 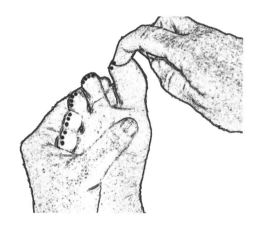

Helper reflexes- Endocrine glands for hormone imbalances.

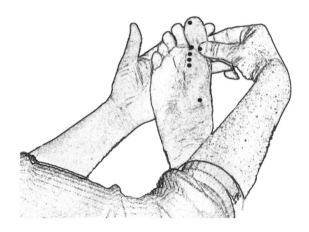 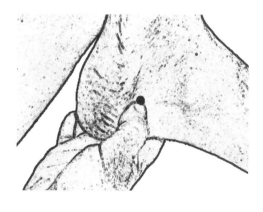

Eyes- for eye strain.

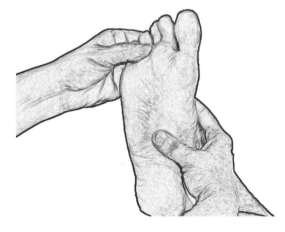 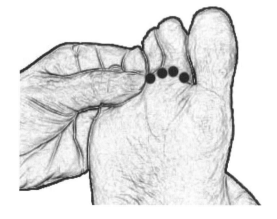

Sinuses- to help with drainage.

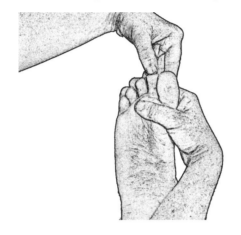 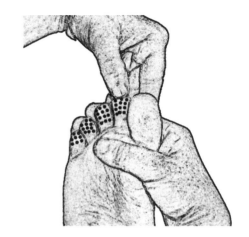

Solar plexus- to relax the body.

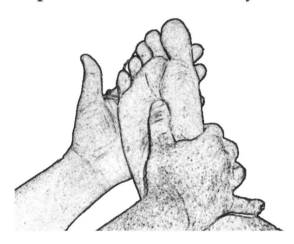 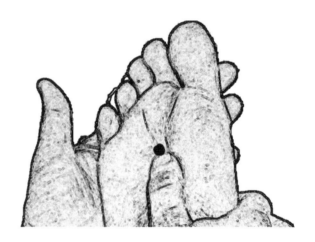

Whole Spine- the neck is usually the culprit, work the whole spine to balance.

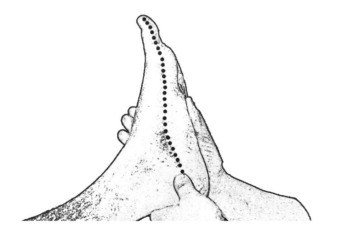 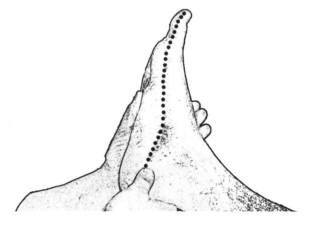

A herniated and ruptured disc is when the soft part between the disc presses on the nerves.

Direct reflex- Spine work the affected area.

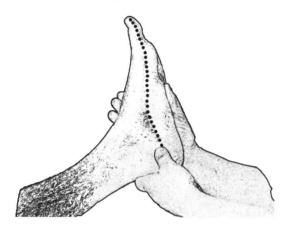 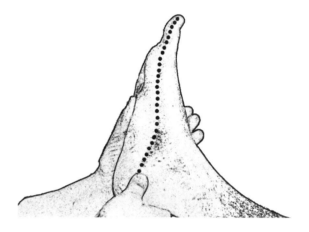

Helper Reflexes- Adrenal for inflammation.

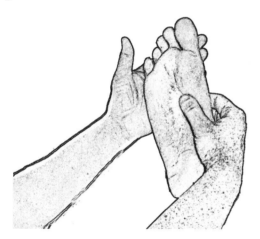 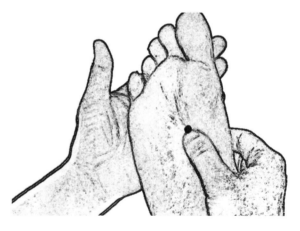

Solar plexus for tension from pain.

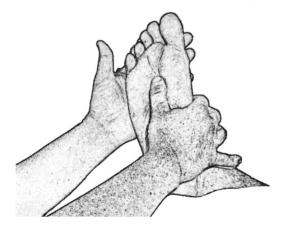 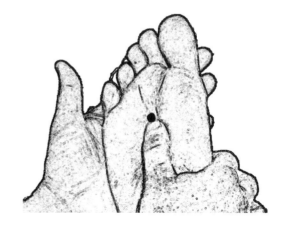

A migraine is caused by vascular irregularities; the altering constriction and expansion of the arteries of the head exerts pressure on the arterial nerves and cause sharp pain.

Direct reflex- Brain

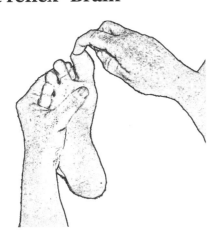
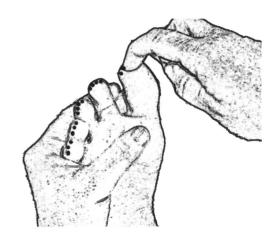

Helper Reflexes- Sinuses to help with drainage.

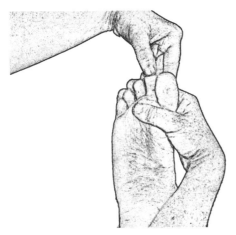
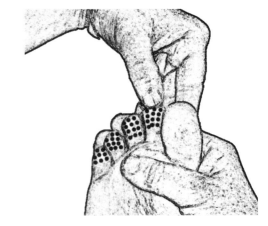

Jaw for TMJ to help relax the jaw.

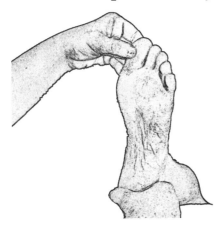
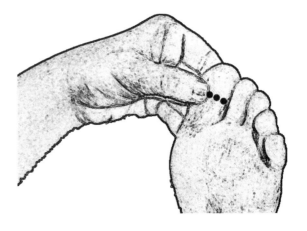

Endocrine glands for hormone imbalances.

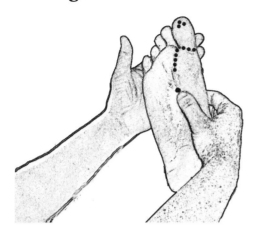 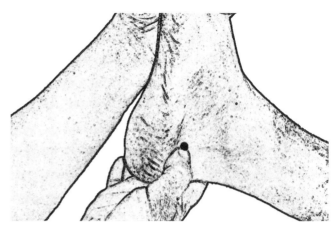

Solar Plexus relieves stress and tension.

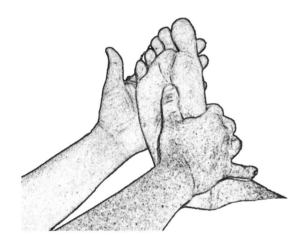 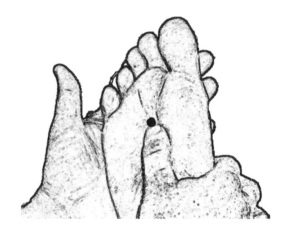

Multiple Sclerosis is a disabling disease of the central nervous system. Sclerosis means scars; these are plaques in the brain and spinal cord. In MS, the myelin covering of the nerve fibers is damaged. Inflammation and loss of the myelin causes disruption to the nerve transmission and affects every organ and gland functions of the body.

Direct reflex- Brain and whole spine.

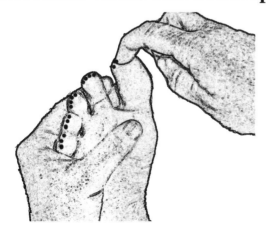 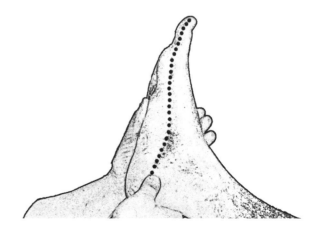

Helper Reflexes- Adrenal for inflammation.

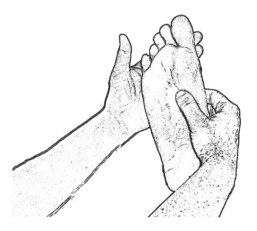 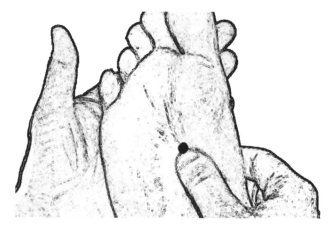

Solar plexus to help with stress and tension.

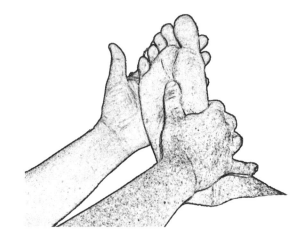 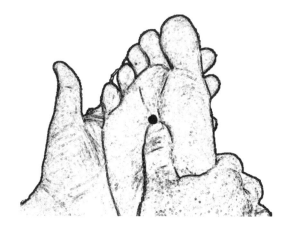

All Systems of the Body to aid in better blood supply throughout the body.

Neck and Back pain- there is a number of underlying reasons for neck and back pain.

Direct reflex- Cervical for neck; **Spine** for back.

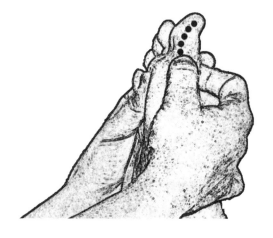 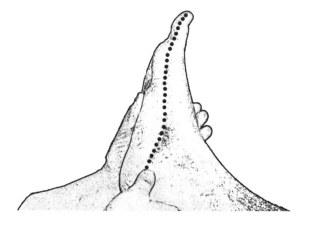

Helper reflexes- Adrenal for inflammation.

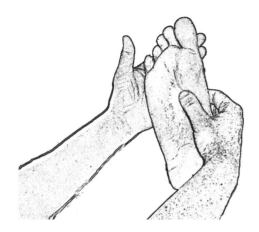 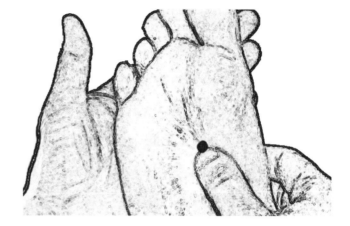

Paralysis loss of voluntary muscular movement.

Direct reflex- Brain

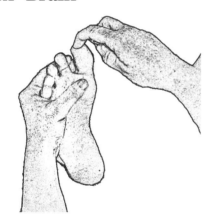 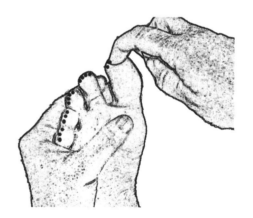

Helper reflexes- Great toe for better blood supply to the brain.

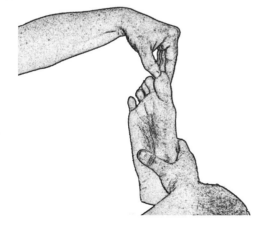 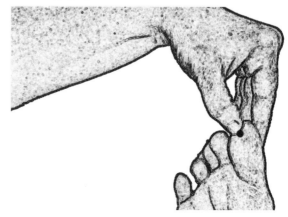

Whole spine for better blood and nerve supply.

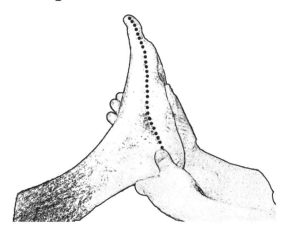 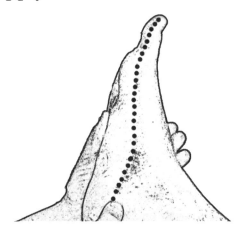

Parkinson's disease it is a progressive loss of function of the nerve cells in the part of the brain that controls muscle movement. Tremors are a result of damaged nerve cells.

Direct reflex- Brain

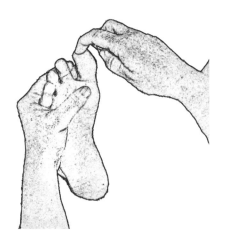 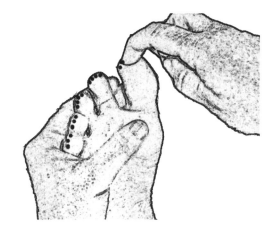

Helper reflexes- Great toe for the brain.

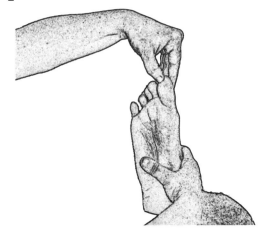 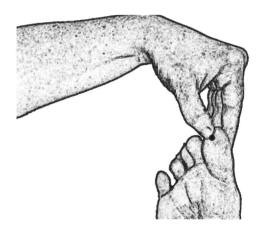

Whole Spine to help revitalizing the Central Nervous System.

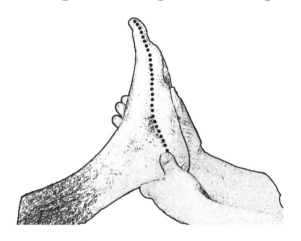 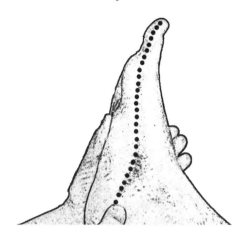

Sciatica pain in the sciatic nerve, usually from a lower disc in the spine pressing on the sciatic nerve.

Direct reflex- Sciatic nerve

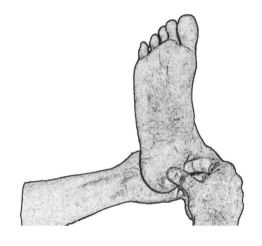 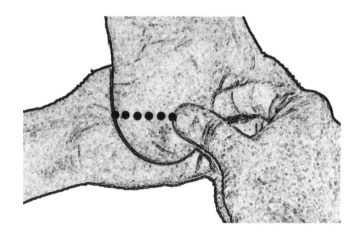

Helper Reflexes- Lumbar for better nerve supply.

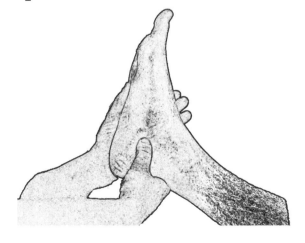 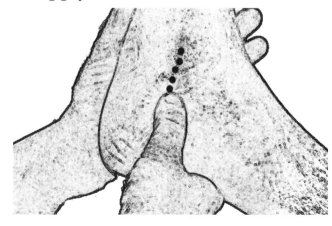

Sacral/Coccyx for better nerve supply.

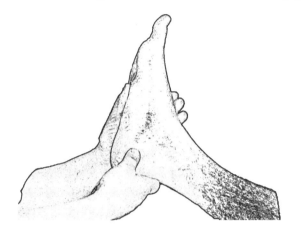
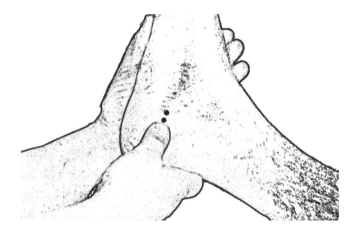

Adrenal for inflammation.

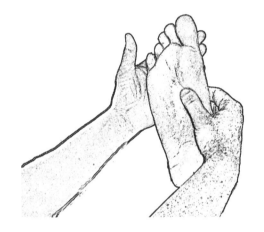
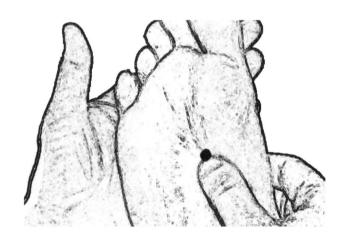

Stroke occurs when part of the brain is damaged because of the blood supply being disturbed.

Direct reflex- Brain

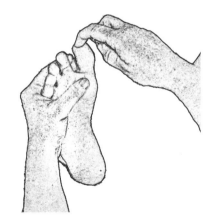
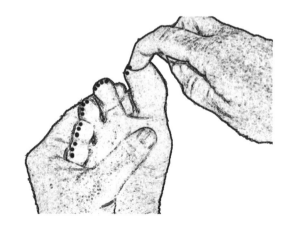

Helper reflexes- Great toes for better blood and nerve supply.

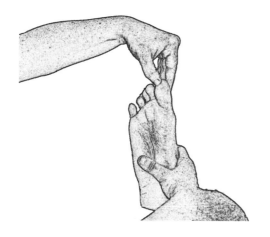 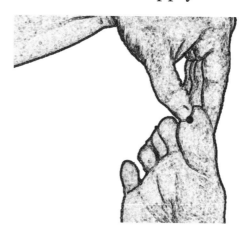

Spine for better blood and nerve supply.

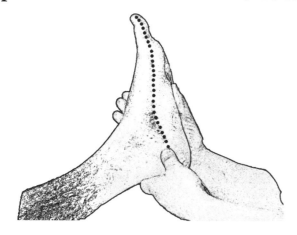 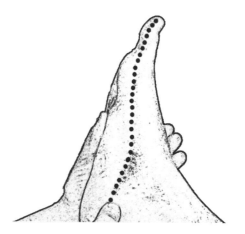

Whiplash is a sudden movement of the head that can lead to tearing muscles, ligaments, and other soft tissue.

Direct Reflex- All neck reflexes for better nerve supply.

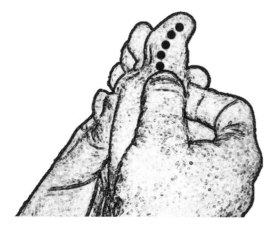 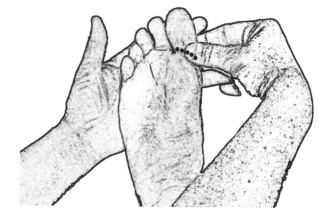

Helper Reflexes- Adrenal for inflammation.

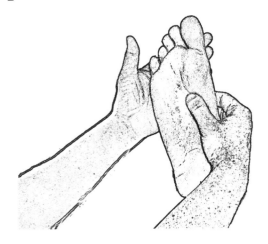
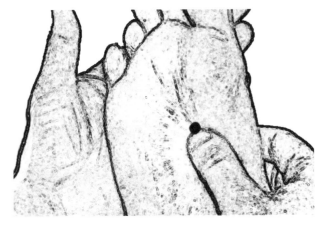

Thoracic for better blood and nerve supply.

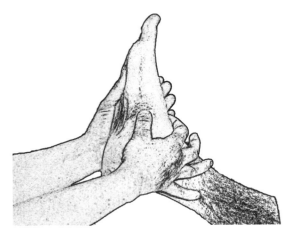
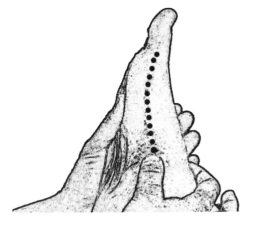

Quiz on the Central Nervous System

1. The cerebrum is located where?
   A) upper part of the forebrain   B) base of the forebrain
   C) deep in the forebrain

2. The cerebellum is located where?
   A) above the spinal cord   B) between the medulla and the midbrain
   C) rear of the brain stem

3. Where is the brain reflex located?
   A) one-quarter inch down from the tip of the great toe
   B) tip of each toe   C) the base line of the great toe

4. How many peripheral nerves exit the spinal cord?
   A) 34   B) 32   C) 31

5. The first cervical peripheral nerve leads to where?
   A) eyes   B) head, pituitary   C) neck, shoulders

6. The second thoracic peripheral nerve leads to where?
   A) lungs , breast, chest   B) stomach   C) heart

7. The third lumbar peripheral nerve leads to where?
   A) large colon   B) reproductive, bladder   C) lower legs

8. Where is the spinal reflex located?
   A) lateral side of the foot   B) medial side of the foot   C) plantar

9. The sciatic nerve begins where in the body?
   A) lumbar region   B) sacral   C) coccyx

10. Where is the sciatic nerve reflex located?
    A) center plantar part of the heel   B) medial below the heel line
    C) lateral part at the heel line

* Answer key on page 325

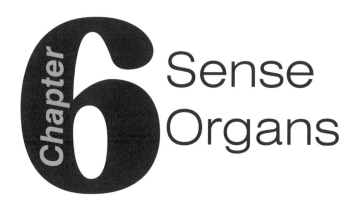

Chapter 6

Sense Organs

Sense Organs

The **Eyes** are the most important of the senses. Your eyes tell you more than the other senses do, and the part of the brain that deals with sight is far larger than the parts that deal with the other senses. This is a guide to the many parts of the eye and how they function:

Sclera- is the white of the eye and it is the protective outer cover. There are six tiny muscles that connect to it and control eye movement.

Iris- is the colored part of the eye. It is able to expand and reduce the size of the pupil.

Cornea- is the opaque water-like fluid in front of the eyeball that has two purposes: protecting the eye and breaking up light as it enters the eye.

Pupil- is the opening of the eye in the center of the iris. It allows light to enter the eye and be absorbed by the retina.

Lens- provides object distance, image distance and focal length.

Conjunctiva- is a transparent tissue that covers the outer surface of the eye. It is nourished by tiny blood vessels.

Vitreous- is a transparent substance that fills the center of the eye. It helps to give it form.

Choroid- is the layers of blood vessels that nourish the back of the eye.

Optic Nerve- is on the very back of the eyeball. Rays of light are converted to electrical impulses from the retina then through the optic nerve that sends impulses to the brain.

Macula- is located in the center of the retina. It is responsible for central vision, such as reading.

Retina- is the inner surface that contains rods and cones, which detects frequency of incoming light.

The reflex areas are on the plantar part of both feet in Zones 2 & 3 at the plantar part between the middle phalanges and proximal phalanges (under second & third small toes). Thumb-walk this area.

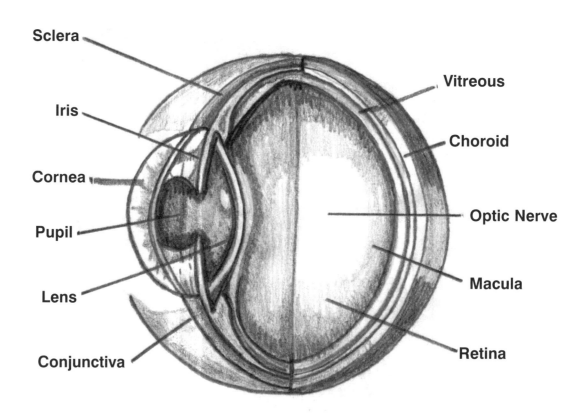

The **Ear** consists of three parts: outer ear, middle ear, and the inner ear. The outer and middle ear are the mechanism for transmission of sound. The inner ear analyzes sound waves and it also contains the mechanism by which the body keeps balance.

OUTER EAR:

Auricle- is the visible part of the ear.

Ear canal- is about one inch long.

MIDDLE EAR:

Ear drum- it receives and transmit sound waves.

Hammer- it joins the inside of the ear drum. Vibrations are transmitted here.

Anvil- it has one broad joint, vibrations are transmitted here.

Stirrup- a delicate bone, vibrations are transmitted here.

Eustachian Tube- this tube connects the inner cavity of the ear with the throat and it equalizes air pressure on both sides of the ear drum.

INNER EAR:

Vestibule- helps control your sense of balance.

Semicircular Canals- sense of motion.

Cochlea- contains hearing nerves. It is a tubular bone that looks like a snail and is about the size of a pea.

The reflex areas are located on both plantar (bottom) part of the feet in Zones 4 & 5 between the middle phalanges and proximal phalanges (under the fourth & fifth small toes). Thumb-walk these areas.

Diagram of the Ear

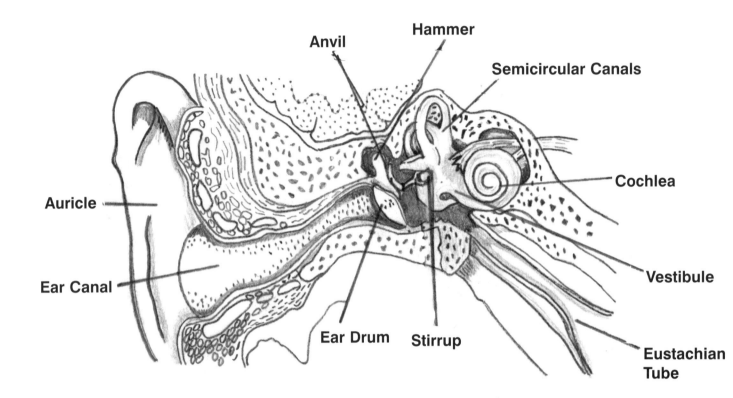

Locate the Reflex areas of the Sense Organs

*Use colored pencils to draw in reflex areas

    A) Ears

    B) Eyes

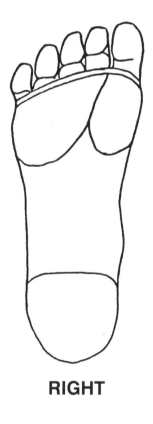

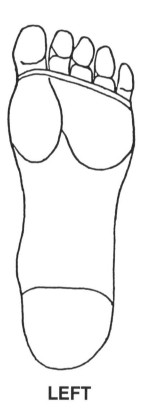

RIGHT   **LEFT**

*Answer key on next page

Answer Key to the Sense Reflex Areas

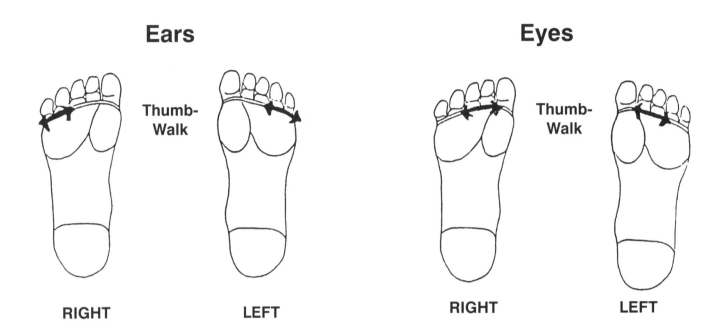

Ears

Thumb-Walk

RIGHT   LEFT

Eyes

Thumb-Walk

RIGHT   LEFT

How to Work the Sense Organ Reflex Areas

The **Ear reflex areas** are on both feet at the baseline of the toes, in Zones 4-5. Thumb-walk these areas.

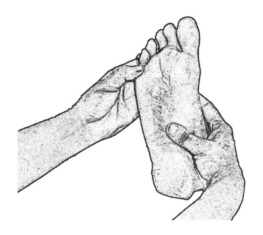
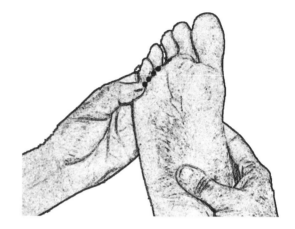

The **Eye reflex areas** are on both feet at the baseline of the toes, in Zones 2-3. Thumb-walk these areas.

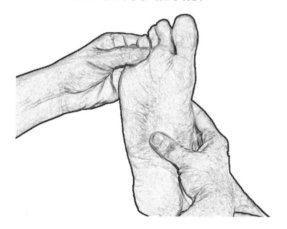
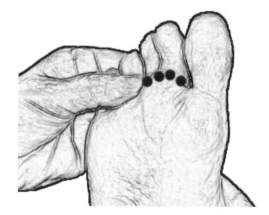

Ear Disorders and the Helper Reflex Areas

Ear Infection- is inflammation in the outer to middle ear and can produce severe pain.

Direct Reflex- Ears for inflammation.

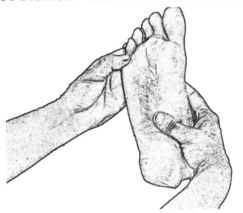 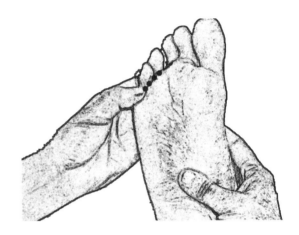

Helper Reflexes- Adrenal for the inflammation.

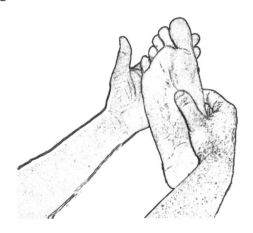 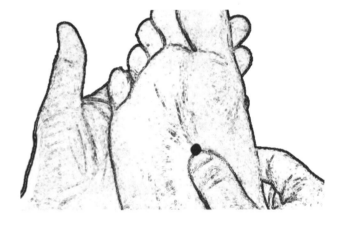

Lymphatic system for infection.

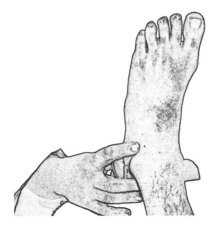 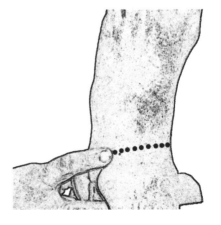

Kidneys to help flush impurities out of the system.

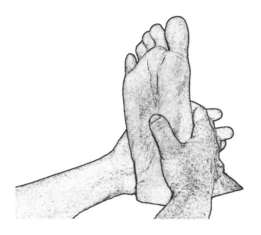 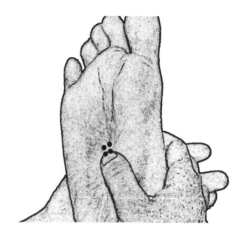

1-4 Cervical the peripheral nerve that leads to the ears.

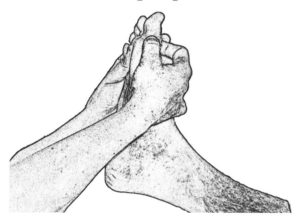 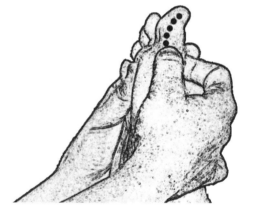

Liver to detoxify.

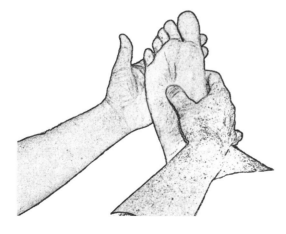 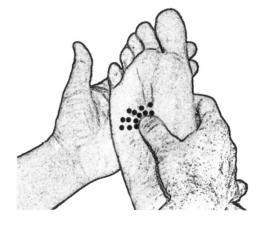

Tinnitus- is noise in the ear. The noise may be a buzzing, ringing, roaring, or hissing. It could be caused from anemia, high blood pressure, low thyroid hormone levels, or from a head injury.

Direct Reflex- Ears

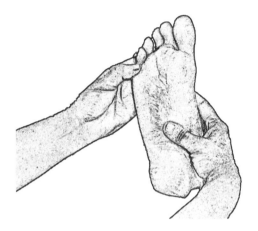 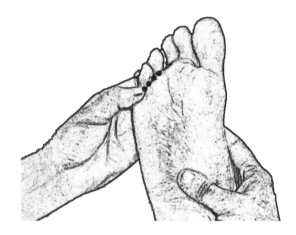

Helper Reflexes- Adrenal control blood volume and pressure.

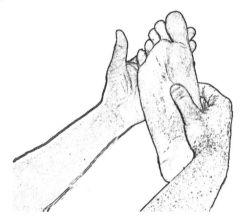 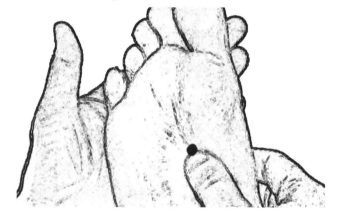

Thyroid to stimulate thyroid levels.

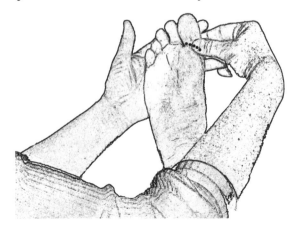 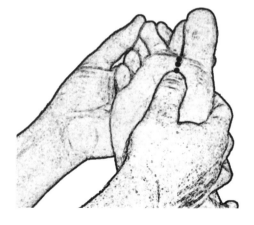

Pituitary for high blood pressure.

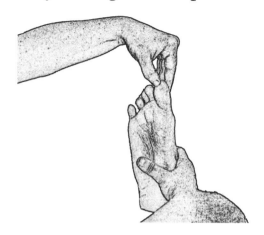 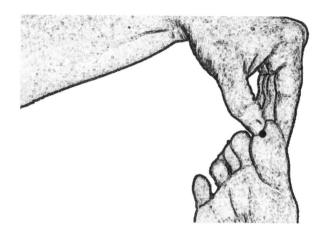

1-4 Cervical the peripheral nerves lead to the ear.

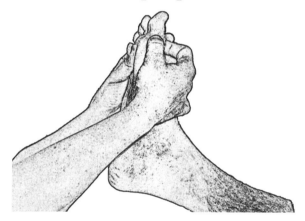 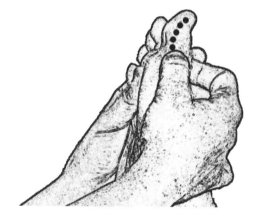

Spleen if it is caused by anemia.

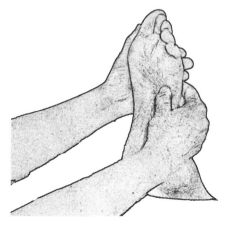 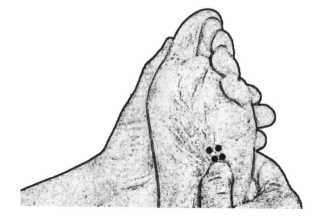

Vertigo- is a loss of balance, dizziness, or a feeling of as if the room is spinning. It is usually a symptom of a disorder of the inner ear, the part of the ear that senses movement and maintains balance.

Direct Reflex- Ear

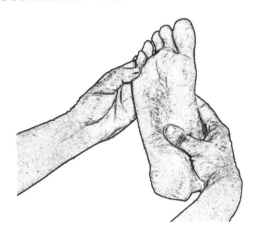 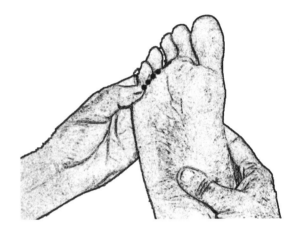

Helper Reflexes- Adrenal for inflammation.

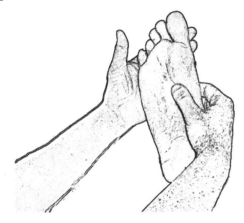 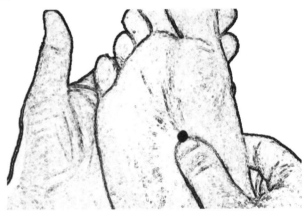

Great toe for everything in the head region.

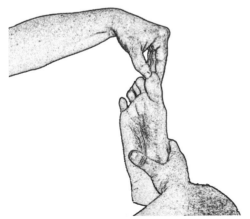 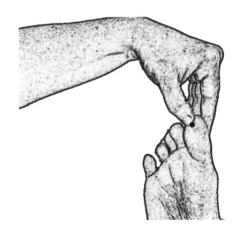

1-4 Cervical the peripheral nerve that leads to the ear.

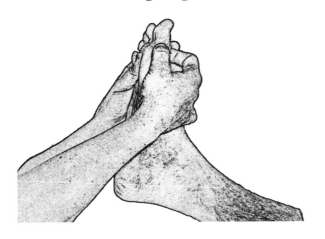 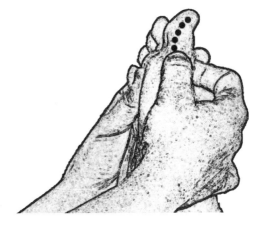

Sinuses to help with drainage.

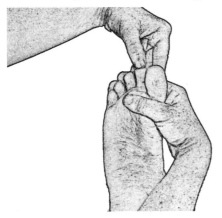 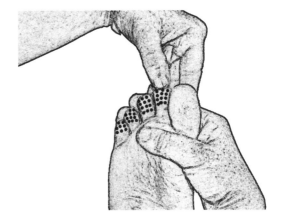

Eye Disorders and the Helper Reflex Areas

Cataracts- is a opaque film that develops in the eyes, causing blurred vision. It is a clouding of the lens.

Direct Reflex- Eyes

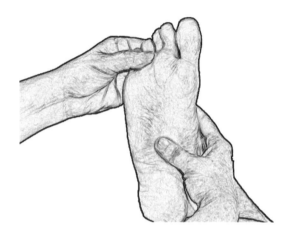
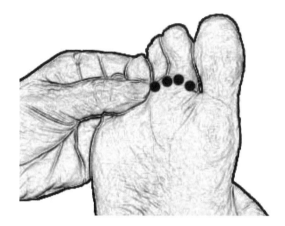

Helper Reflexes- Kidneys, as they regulate the retention of water.

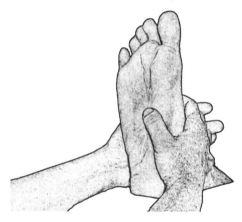
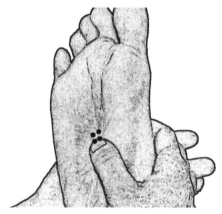

Pituitary for fluid retention.

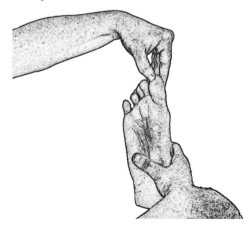
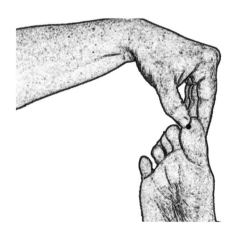

2nd Cervical the peripheral nerve that leads to the eye.

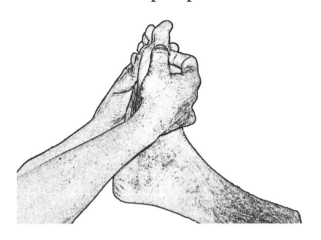 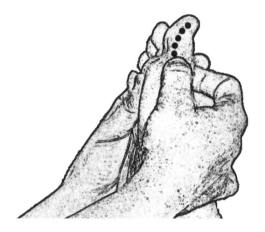

Glaucoma- is a malfunction of the eye's drainage structures and causes pressure by excess fluid in the eye.

Direct Reflex- Eye

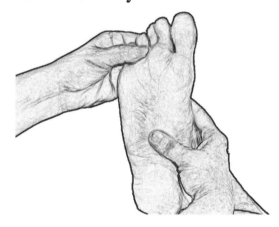 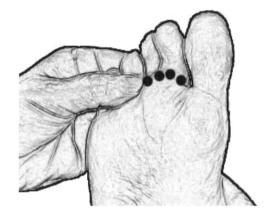

Helper Reflexes- Kidneys for fluid retention.

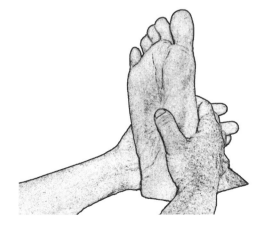 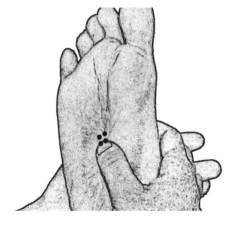

Pituitary for fluid retention.

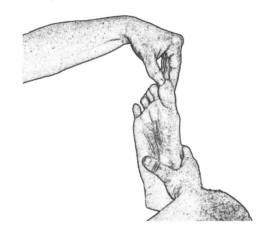 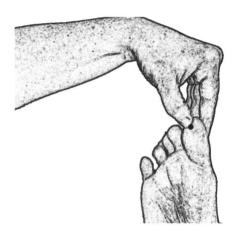

2nd Cervical the peripheral nerve that leads to the eye.

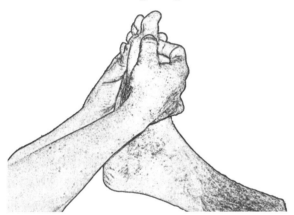 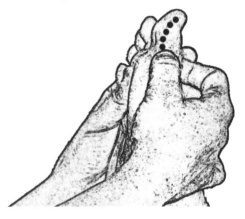

Macular Degeneration- is usually age related. It is a degeneration of the macula. It is caused by hardening of the arteries that nourish the retina. This takes away from the sensitive retinal tissue the oxygen and nutrients that it needs to function. The outcome is that the central vision deteriorates.

Direct Reflex- Eye

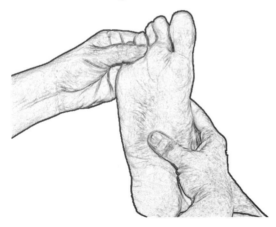 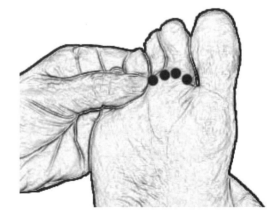

Helper Reflexes- Kidney for fluid retention.

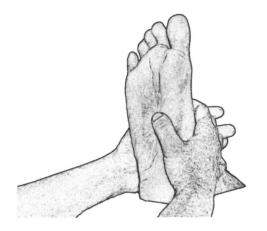 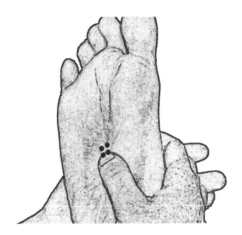

Pituitary for fluid retention.

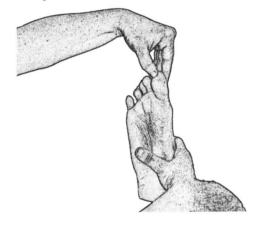 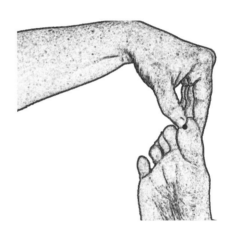

2nd Cervical the peripheral nerve that leads to the eye.

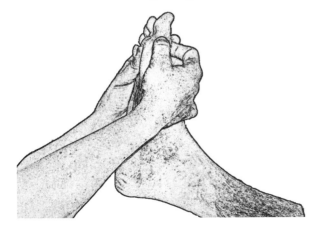 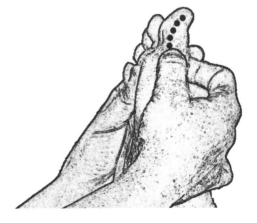

Retinopathy- occurs when diabetes damages the tiny vessels in the retina. The arteries in the retina becomes weak and leak causing small hemorrhages. These leaking vessels often lead to swelling in the retina and decrease the vision.

Direct Reflex- Eyes

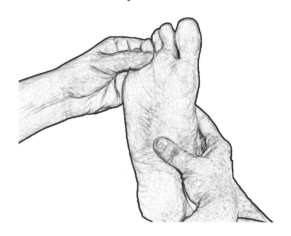
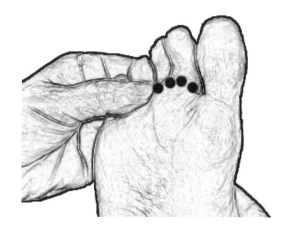

Helper Reflexes- Pancreas to help fluid retention.

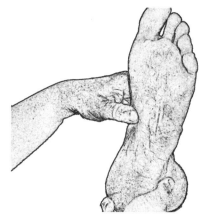
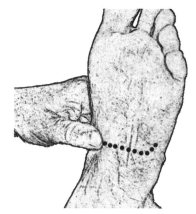

Adrenal for inflammation.

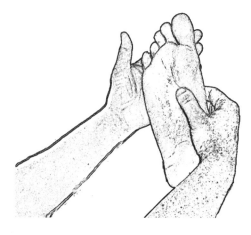
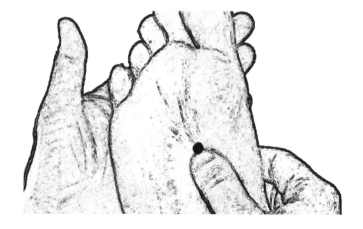

Pituitary to regulate fluid retention.

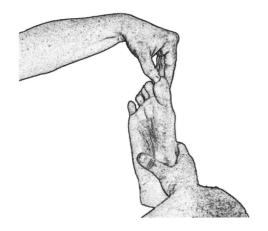 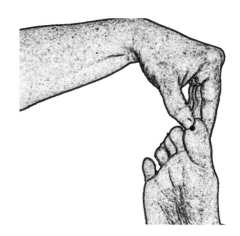

Kidneys to regulate fluid retention.

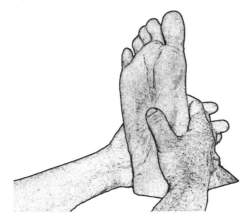 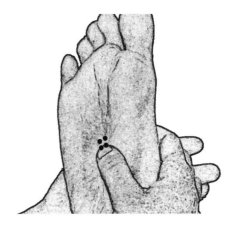

2nd Cervical the peripheral nerve lead to the eye.

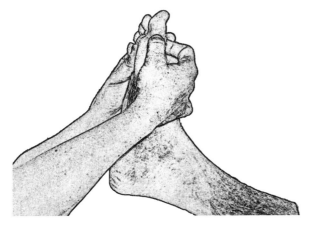 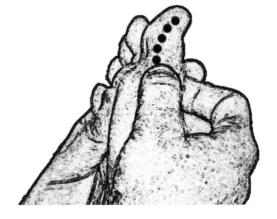

Quiz on the Sense Organs

1. What part of the eye is the Iris?

   A) white outer cover B) colored part C) the opening in the center

2. What part of the eye is the Sclera?

   A) white outer cover

   B) the opaque water-like fluid in front of the eyeball C) colored part

3. Where is the optic nerve located in the eye?

   A) the very back of, the eyeball

   B) the center of the retina C) the inner surface

4. Where are the eye reflex areas located?

   A) under the fourth & fifth toes

   B) under the second & third toes C) the tip of the second & third toes

5. The Auricle is what part of the ear? A) inner B) outer C) middle

6. The Vestibule does what? A) receives and transmit sound waves

   B) controls sense of balance C) vibrations are transmitted here

7. The Anvil is what part of the ear? A) inner B) middle C) outer

8. Where are the ear reflex areas located?

   A) under the second & third toes B) under the fourth & fifth

   C) tip of the fourth & fifth toes

*Answer key on page 325

Chapter 7

Endocrine System

The Endocrine System

The Endocrine glands produce hormones that travel directly into the bloodstream. These glands regulate the body's activities such as growth, sleep, emotions, and quick actions. The Endocrine glands are located in different parts of the body.

- Hypothalamus, pituitary, and pineal are in the brain
- Thyroid and Parathyroid are in the neck
- Adrenal are above the kidneys
- Islands of Langerhans are in the pancreas
- Ovaries and testes (reproductive) are in the lower abdomen

The Adrenal are small triangular glands located on top of the kidneys. They have over fifty functions. The adrenal work with the hypothalamus and pituitary. Adrenal have two parts consisting of the, adrenal cortex and adrenal medulla. **The Adrenal Cortex** is the outer part of the gland. It is essential to life since it secretes hormones and promotes metabolism by controlling energy levels.

The adrenal cortex secrete corticosteroids and other hormones directly into the bloodstream:

- Hydrocortisone hormone- controls the body's use of fats, proteins, and carbohydrates
- Cortisterone- this hormone with the hydrocortisone hormones, suppresses inflammatory reactions of the body and affects the immune system
- Aldosterone hormone- controls the level of sodium excreted into the urine, controlling the blood volume and pressure
- Androgenic steroids- these hormones have a small effect on development of male characteristics.

The Adrenal Medulla is the inner part of the gland. It helps with physical and emotional stress, and secretes adrenaline:
- Adrenaline- this hormone increases heart rate, facilitates blood flow to the brain and muscles, relaxes the smooth muscles, and helps with the conversion of glycogen to glucose in the liver.

The Adrenal reflex area is found on both feet on the plantar (bottom) side between Zones 1 and 2 about one-half inch down from the diaphragm line. Thumb-walk these areas.

Hypothalamus- is located in the brain. The main function is homeostasis. It helps to regulate body temperature, control blood pressure, heart rate, food and water intake, and metabolism of fats, carbohydrates, and sugar levels in the blood. The role of the hypothalamus is the expression of emotions, such as pleasure, pain fear, and sexual behavior.

The hormones the hypothalamus releases are:
• Thyrotropin (TRH)
• Gonadotropin (GnRH)
• Growth hormone (GHRH)
• Ghrelin
• Corticotropin (CRH)
• Somatostin
• Dopamine

These hormones are released into the bloodstream and travel to the Anterior Lobe of the pituitary.

The reflex area is found on both feet on the plantar (bottom) part of the great toe about one-quarter inch down from the tip of the great toe. Reflex with one thumb-press.

Pineal Gland- is a small organ about the size of a pea. Which is located in the brain. The Pineal produces the hormone Melatonin, which regulates the body rhythms. Melatonin is released during sleep.

The reflex areas are found in both feet on the plantar (bottom) part of the great toe. It is about one-quarter down from the tip of the great toe. Reflex with one thumb-press.

Pituitary Gland- is a peanut size organ situated beneath the brain. It is often called the master gland, controlling the secretion of almost every hormone in the body. To name a few of its activities: it affects sexual development, fever, fainting, metabolism, mineral and sugar contents of the blood, fluid retention, and energy levels. The Pituitary is attached to the Hypothalamus by nerve fibers. The Pituitary consists of three sections:

- Anterior Lobe
- Intermediate Lobe
- Posterior Lobe

Functions of the Pituitary gland:

Anterior Lobe:

- growth hormone
- prolactin- to stimulate milk production after giving birth
- ACHT (Adrenocricotropic) stimulate adrenal glands
- FSH (follicle-stimulating hormone) stimulate ovary and testes
- TSH (thyroid stimulating hormone) stimulate thyroid
- LH (luteinizing hormone) stimulate ovaries and testes

Intermediate Lobe:

- Melanogte- stimulating hormone to control skin pigmentation

Posterior Lobe:

- ADH (anti-diuretic hormone) to increase the absorption of water into the blood by the kidneys, and oxytocin to contract the uterus during childbirth and stimulate milk production.

The reflex areas are on both feet on the plantar (bottom) part of the great toe, about one-quarter down from the tip of the great toe. Reflex with one thumb-press.

The **Thyroid**, the largest gland in the neck, is butterfly shaped and located in the lower anterior part of the neck.The function is to make the thyroid hormone called thyroxine, which regulates the body's metabolism, organ function, heart rate, cholesterol level, body weight, energy level, muscle strength, skin condition, memory, and menstrual regularity. The thyroid influences every organ, tissue, and cell in the body.

The reflex is found on both feet on the plantar (bottom) part at the base of the great toe and between the 1st and 2nd metatarsal. Thumb-walk these reflexes.

The **Parathyroids** are located on the four corners of the thyroid gland. There are four parathyroid glands. The glands produce the parathyroid hormone.

The parathyroid hormone stimulates the following functions:
- release of calcium by bones into the blood stream
- absorption of food by the intestines
- conservation of calcium by the kidneys

The reflex areas are found on both feet on the plantar (bottom) part of the base of the great toe and between the 1st and 2nd metatarsal. Thumb-walk these reflexes.

The Islands of Langerhans- (endocrine pancreas) are located in the pancreas. They secrete the hormones glucagon and insulin and they are scattered throughout the pancreas. Their purpose is to make insulin in the correct amount in the right time.

Islets means "little islands" because of the clusters in the pancreas. Islets are made up mostly of beta cells that make insulin. There is a few alpha cells and delta cells, which have important roles in changing food to energy.

Hormone secreted by pancreatic islets cells:

• **Insulin**	beta cells	lowers blood sugar
• **Glucagon**	alpha cells	raises blood sugar
• **Somatostatin**	delta cells	inhibits insulin, glucagon, PP, and exocrine pancreas
• **Pancreatic Polypeptide (PP)**	F cell	stimulates pepsin and HCI (acid) secretion by stomach.

The reflex areas are found on both feet on the plantar (bottom) part of the foot on the right foot, in Zone 1 near the 1st cuneiform. On the left foot it's in Zones 1-4 across the 1st-3rd cuneiforms. Thumb-walk these reflex areas.

Ovary- secretes the hormone estrogen and progesterone. These hormones control the development of female sexual features such as breast and growth of the body's fat around the hips and thighs. These hormones are involved in pregnancy and the regulation of menstruation.

Testes- secrete hormones called androgens, the most important of which is testosterone. These hormones regulate body changes associated with sexual development, height, change in the voice (getting deeper), growth of facial hair and pubic hair, increased muscle growth and strength.

The reflex areas are located on the lateral (outside) part of both feet between the talus (ankle) and the calcaneous (heel). On the diagonal from the back of the heel to the ankle bone, it is at the halfway mark. Thumb-press this area.

* A diagram of the Endocrine System is the on next page.

Diagram of the Endocrine System

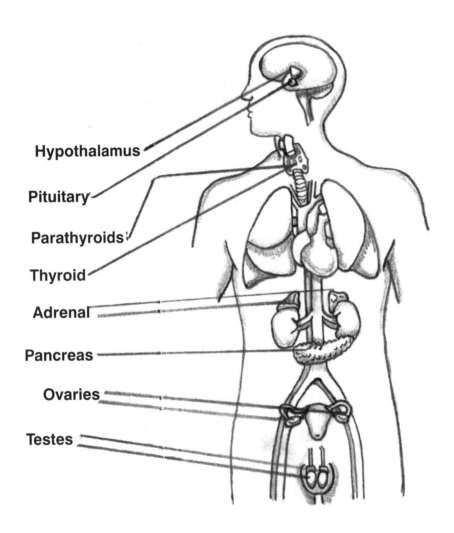

Hypothalamus

Pituitary

Parathyroids

Thyroid

Adrenal

Pancreas

Ovaries

Testes

Locate the Reflex Areas of the Endocrine System

*Use colored pencils to draw in reflex areas

    A) Adrenal

    B) Hypothalamus

    C) Islands of Langerhans

    D) Pineal gland

    E) Pituitary

    F) Thyroid / Parathyroid

    G) Ovary / Testes

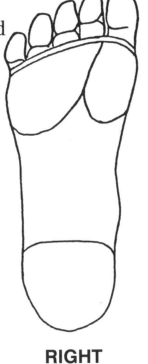
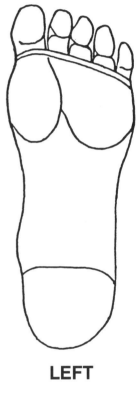

RIGHT   **LEFT**

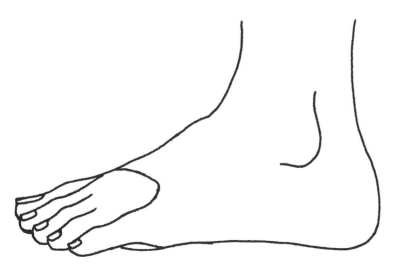

*Answer key on next page

Answer Key to the Endocrine Reflex Areas

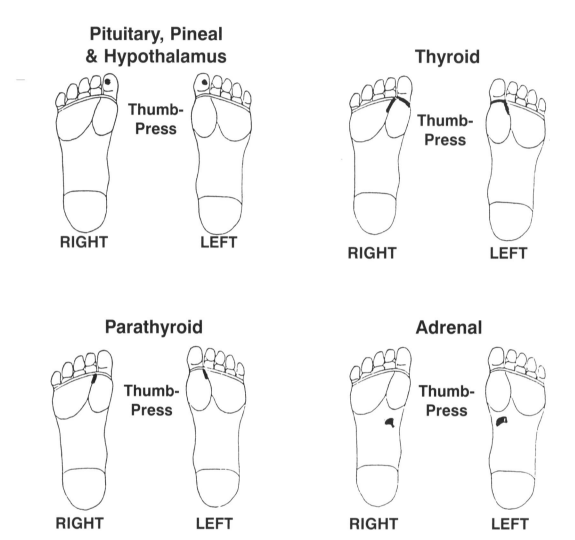

Pituitary, Pineal & Hypothalamus

Thumb-Press

RIGHT   LEFT

Thyroid

Thumb-Press

RIGHT   LEFT

Parathyroid

Thumb-Press

RIGHT   LEFT

Adrenal

Thumb-Press

RIGHT   LEFT

Answer Key to the Endocrine Reflex Areas

Islands of Langerhans

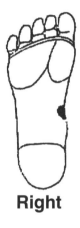 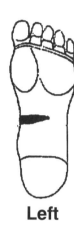

Right   **Left**

Ovary & Testes

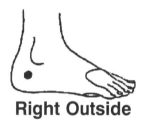

Right Outside

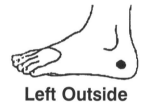

Left Outside

How to Work the Endocrine System Reflex Areas

The **Adrenal reflex areas** are on both feet between Zones 1-2, one inch below the diaphragm line. Thumb-press these areas.

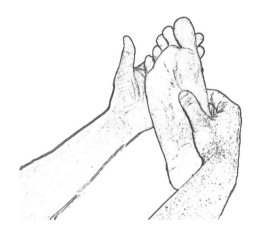
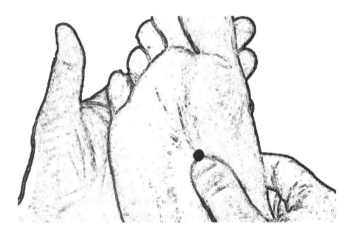

The **Islands of Langerhans (Pancreas) reflex areas** are on both feet; the right foot in Zone 1 at the waistline, and on the left foot it is in Zones 1-4 at the waistline. Thumb-walk these areas.

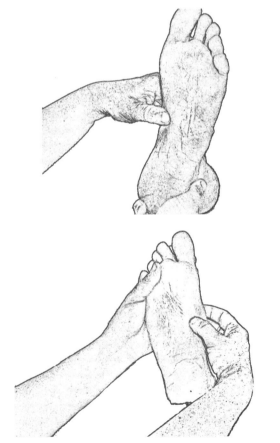
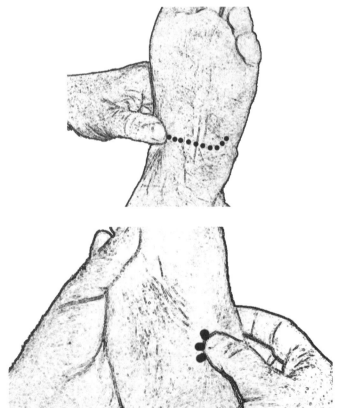

The **Ovary/Testes reflex areas** are on both feet on the lateral (outside) part, between the talus (ankle bone) and back of the calcaneous (heel). Thumb-press these areas.

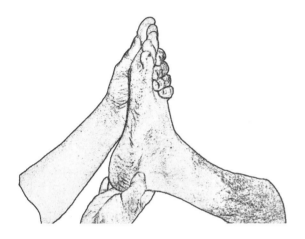
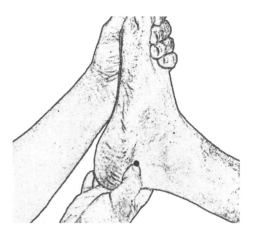

The **Hypothalamus, Pineal, and Pituitary reflex areas** are on both great toes. Thumb-press these areas.

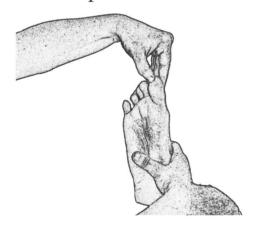
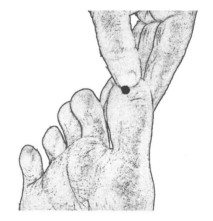

The **Thyroid and Parathyroid reflex areas** are on both feet at the baseline of the great toe and between the first and second metatarsals. Thumb-walk these areas.

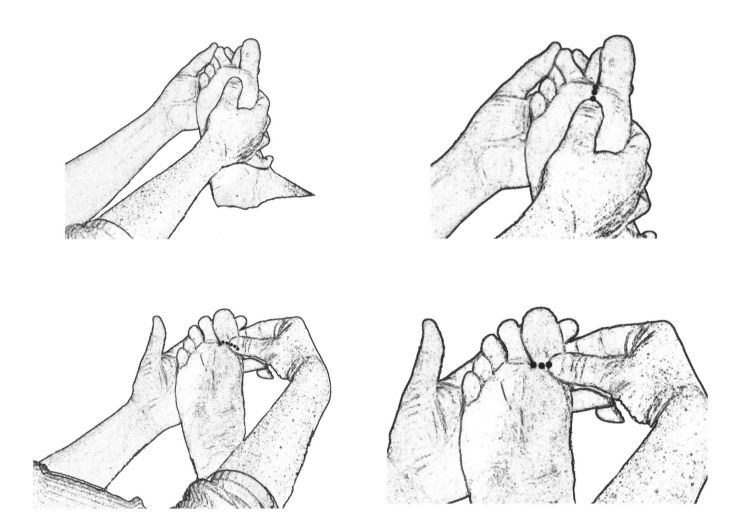

Endocrine Disorders and the Helper Reflex Areas

ADD is a disorder that children are diagnosed with when they have difficulty paying attention, do not listen or follow directions, and are forgetful. Some medical reports believe that the area of the brain is under active.

Direct Reflex- Adrenal- to help with physical and emotional stress.

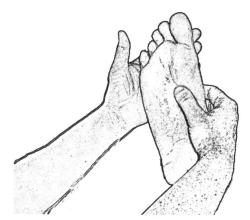 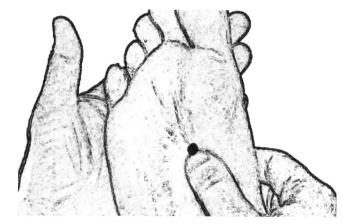

Helper Reflexes- Solar Plexus- to relieve stress and tension.

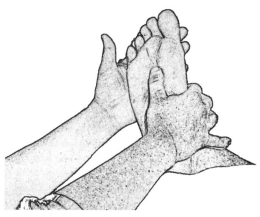 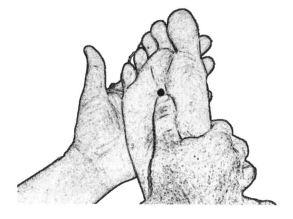

Pituitary- to control energy levels.

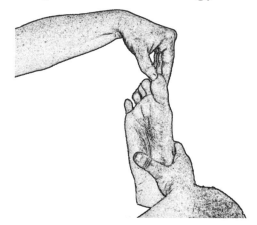 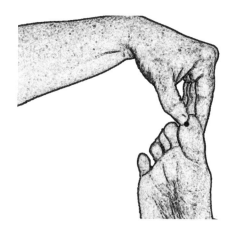

AD/HD is a neurobiological disorder attributed to a deficiency of dopamine.

Direct Reflex- Hypothalamus- to release the hormone dopamine.

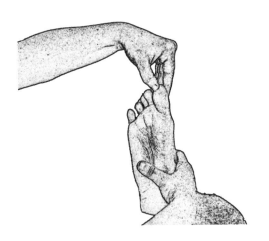 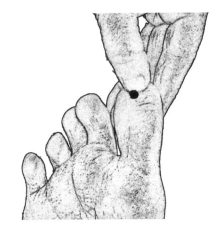

Helper Reflexes- Adrenal- to help with emotional and physical stress.

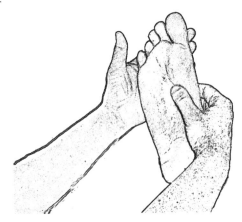 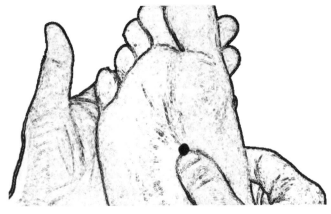

Solar plexus- to help to reduce stress and tension.

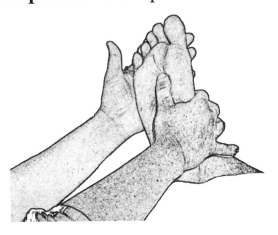 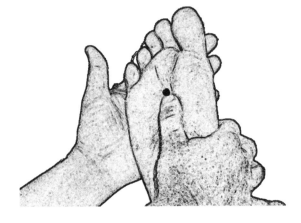

Adrenal Insufficiency is a decreased function of the adrenal cortex.

The adrenal corticosteroid hormone is under produced.

Direct Reflex- Adrenal- to control energy levels.

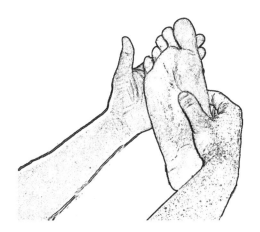 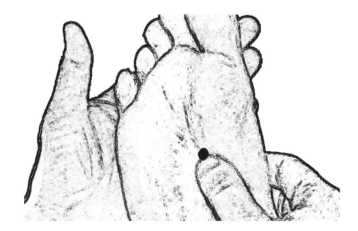

Helper Reflexes- Pituitary- to control secretion of the adrenal hormone.

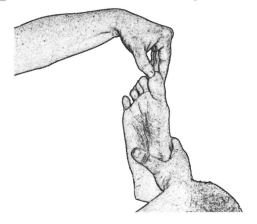 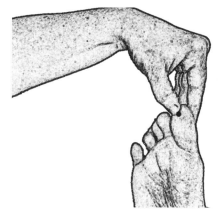

Thyroid- to help control energy levels.

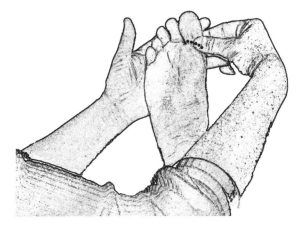 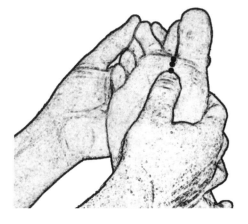

Diabetes (Type1) is when the pancreas fails to produce enough insulin.

Direct Reflex- Pancreas- to help secrete glucagon and insulin.

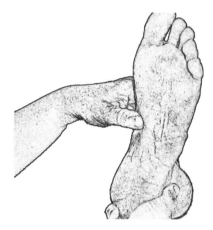 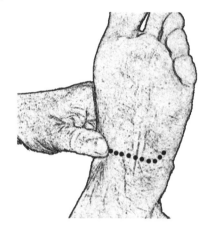

Helper Reflexes- Adrenal- to help with conversion of glycogen to glucose in the liver.

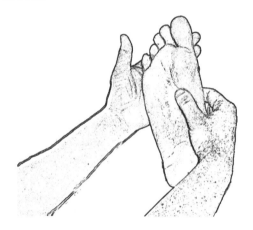 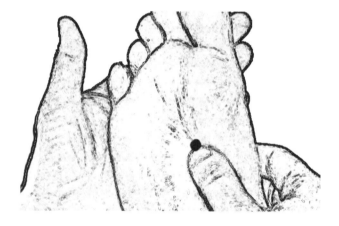

Liver- to regulate the amount of glucose.

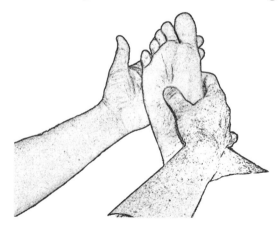 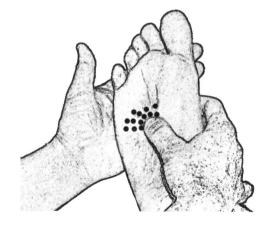

Pituitary- to regulate sugar content in the blood.

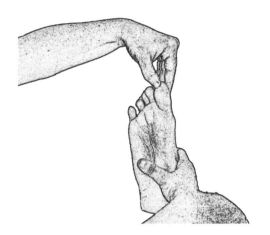
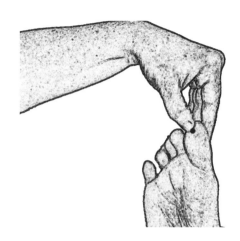

Diabetes (Type 2) unlike Type 1, in which the body can not produce normal amounts of insulin, Type 2 the body is unable to respond to insulin normally. Excess body fat plays a role in the insulin resistance. Look on the internet at www.pacificreflexology.com for all the research studies done on Diabetics.

Direct Reflex- Pancreas- to help secrete glucagon and insulin.

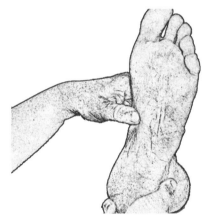
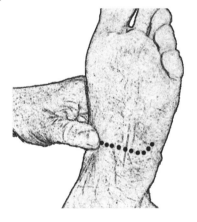

Helper Reflexes- Adrenal- to help with the conversion of glycogen to glucose in the liver.

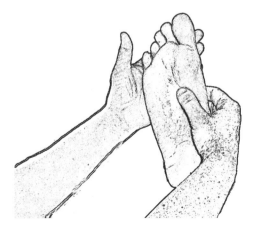
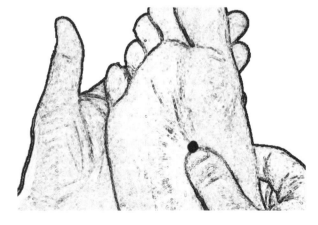

Liver- to regulate the amount of glucose.

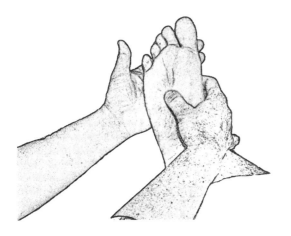 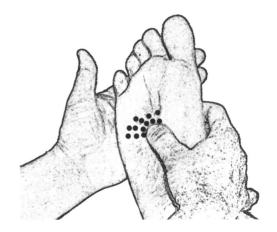

Pituitary- to regulate sugar contents in the blood.

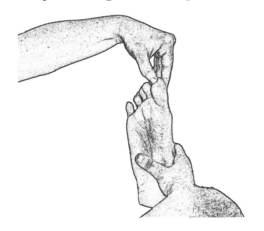 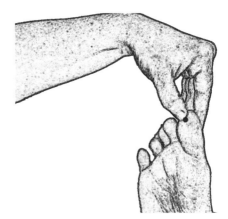

Growth disorders occur when the pituitary gland fails to produce normal amounts of growth hormone, or produces too much growth hormone resulting in gigantism.

Direct Reflex- Pituitary- to regulate the growth hormone.

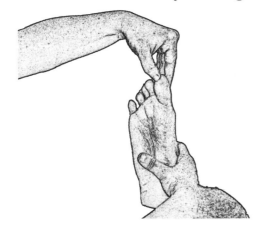 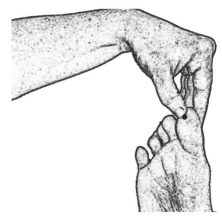

Helper Reflexes- Thyroid- to influence the pituitary.

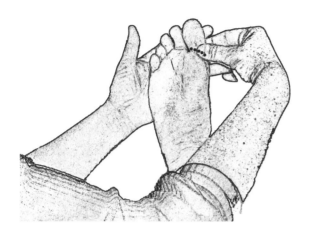 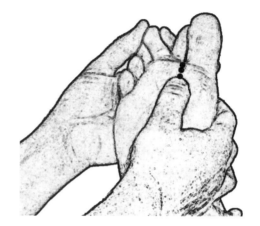

Adrenal- to secrete other hormones into the bloodstream.

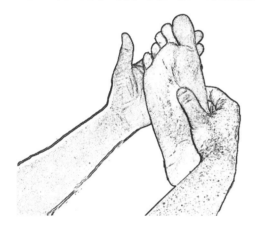 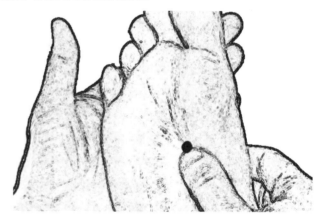

Hypertension (high blood pressure) is the force of the blood flow exerting pressure on the arterial walls.

Direct Reflex- Pituitary- to help control blood pressure.

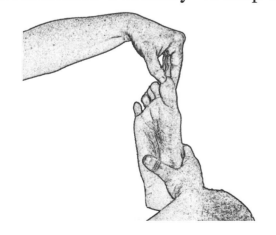 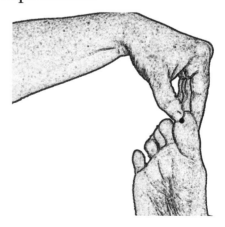

Helper Reflexes- Adrenal- to control blood volume and pressure.

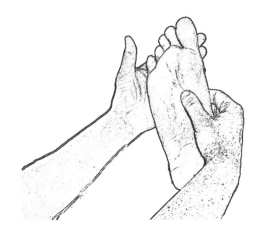 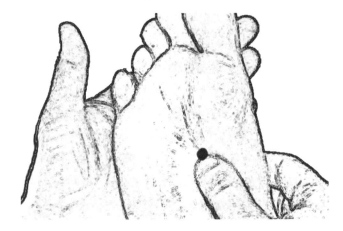

Thyroid- to regulate organ function.

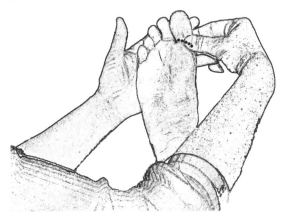 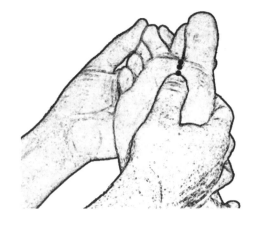

Solar Plexus- to relieve stress and tension.

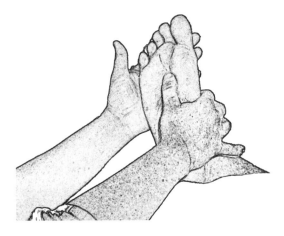 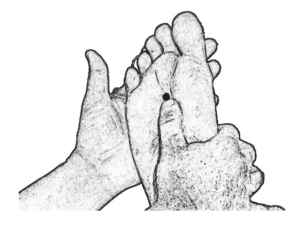

Hyperthyroidism is an excessive production of the thyroid hormone and thyroxine. The symptoms are weight loss, rapid heart rate, nervousness, excessive drinking and urinating.

Direct Reflex- Thyroid- to release thyroxine to regulate the functions.

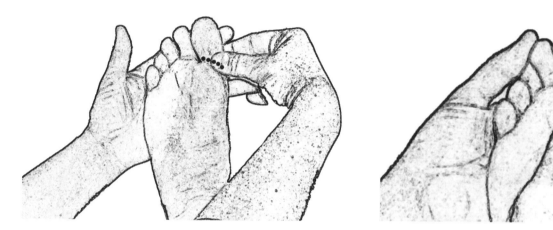

Helper Reflexes- Endocrine glands- to produce hormones into the bloodstream.

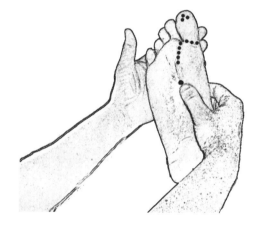
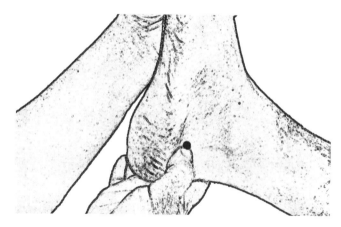

Pituitary- to control secretion of every hormone in the body.

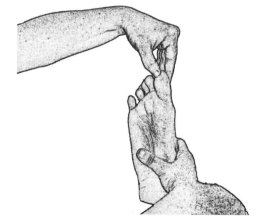
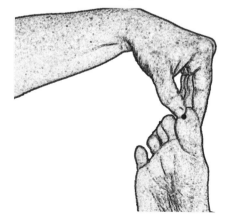

Solar plexus- to relieve stress and tension.

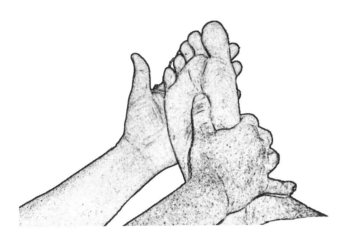 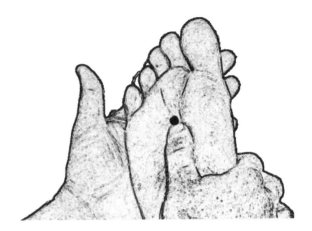

Hypothyroidism is a decreased production of the thyroid hormone thyroxine. The symptoms are weight gain, lethargy, dry skin, and low body temperature.

Direct Reflex- Thyroid- to release thyroxine to regulate the functions.

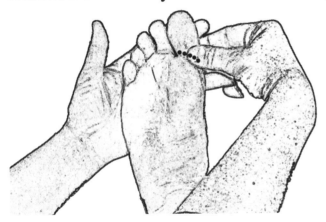 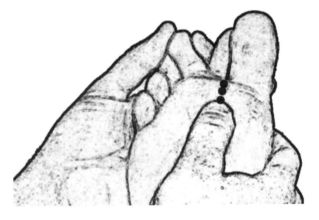

Helper Reflexes- Adrenal- to help with the body's metabolism by controlling the energy levels.

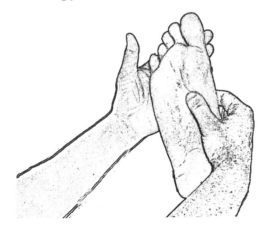 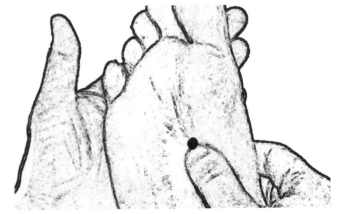

Pituitary- to control secretion of every hormone in the body.

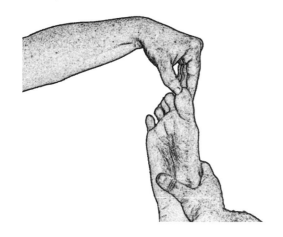 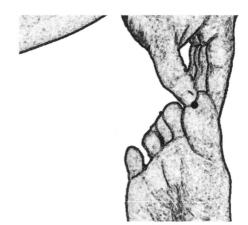

Quiz for the Endocrine System

1. The adrenal are located where in the body?
   A) on top of the gallbladder
   B) on top of the kidneys C) on top of the stomach

2. Which one of the hormones do the adrenal secrete?
   A) Dopamine   B) Melatonin   C) Cortisterone

3. The adrenal are located in which Zone?
   A) 5   B) between 1 & 2   C) 3

4. What is the role of the hypothalamus?
   A) controls blood pressure   B) regulates body rhythms
   C) controls fluid retention

5. Where is the hypothalamus reflex area located?
   A) tips of great toes
   B) one-quarter inch down from the tips of the great toes
   C) medial side of the great toes

6. What hormone does the pineal gland secrete?
   A) growth hormone B) melatonin C) Cortisterone

7. Where is the pineal gland reflex located?
   A) one-quarter inch down the great toe B) tips of all toes
   C) lateral side of the great toe

8. Is the ovary and testes part of the endocrine system?
   A) yes   B) no

9. Where are the ovary and testes reflex areas located?
   A) medial side   B) lateral side C) on the dorsal side

10. How many parathyroid glands are there?
    A) 2   B) 1   C) 4

* Answer key on page 325

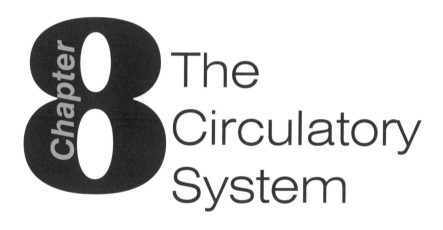

Chapter 8

The Circulatory System

Circulatory System

The Heart is the most vital organ in the circulatory system and is located almost in the center of the chest with two-thirds on the left and one-third on the right. The size of two fists held side-by-side. The heart is the hardest working muscle in the body and is divided into four sections: the right and left ventricle and the right and left atrium. The heart acts like a pump that rhythmically contracts to move five quarts of blood through the vessels in all parts of your body and to bring it back to the heart.

Right & Left Atrium- are the chambers of the heart that receive blood from a vein.

Right & Left Ventricle- are the muscular chambers of the heart that are responsible for pumping blood from the heart into the chambers.

Aortic Valve- opens for the oxygen-rich blood to pass from the left ventricle into the aorta where it travels to the rest of the body.

Mitral Valve- lets oxygen-rich blood pass from the left atrium into the left ventricle.

Pulmonary Valve- controls blood flow from the right ventricle into pulmonary arteries, which carry blood into your lungs to pick up oxygen.

Tricuspid Valve- is between the right atrium and the right ventricle; it regulates the blood flow between them

The Blood Vessels are veins and arteries. They provide the pathway where the blood travels.

Aorta- the largest artery of the body.

Arteries- are muscular blood vessels that carry blood away from the heart.

Arterioles- are small arterial branches that deliver blood into a capillary bed.

Capillaries- carry blood between the smallest arteries and their corresponding veins.

Venules- are small venous branches that carry blood from a capillary to a vein.

Veins- are blood vessels that carry blood to the heart.

Vena Cava- are the two largest veins in the body. They carry deoxygenated blood from the regions of the body to the right atrium.

The reflex areas are found on the plantar (bottom) part of both feet in Zone 1 between the diaphragm line and toe line. Thumb-walk these areas.

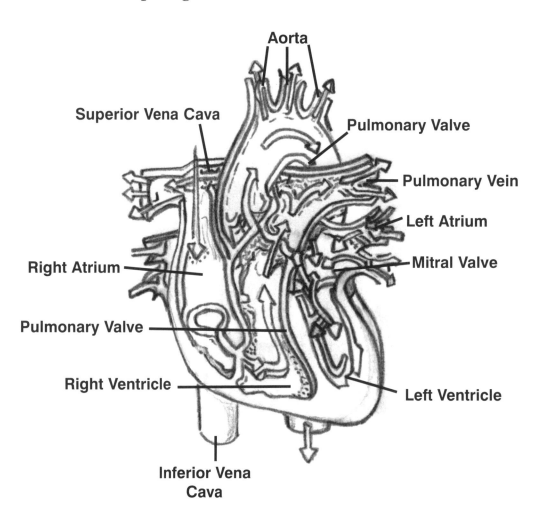

Locate the Reflex Areas of the Heart

*Use colored pencils to draw in reflex areas

A) Heart

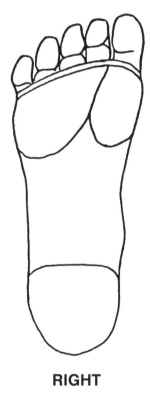

RIGHT

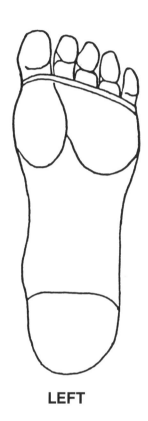

LEFT

*Answer key on next page.

Answer Key for the Heart Reflex

Heart

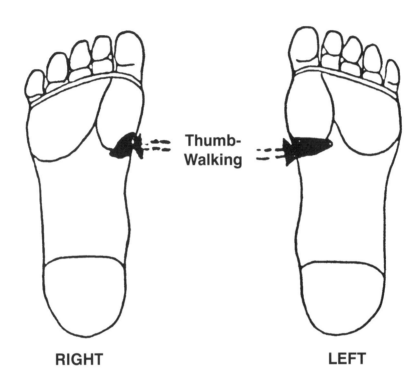

Thumb-Walking

RIGHT   LEFT

How to Work the Heart Reflex Areas

The **Heart reflex areas** are on both feet plantar (bottom) part. In Zone 1 on the diaphragm line on the right foot; on the left foot it is in Zone 1 on the diaphragm line. Thumb-walk these areas.

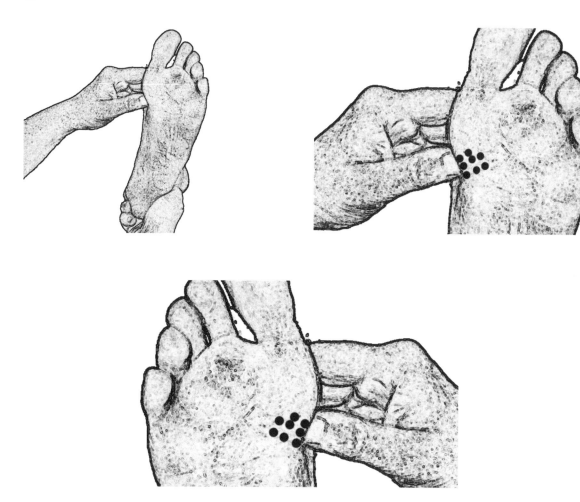

Heart Disorders and the Helper Reflex Areas

Angina Pectoris- is the name for pain that occurs when the muscular wall of the heart becomes temporarily short of oxygen and blood.

Direct Reflex- Heart

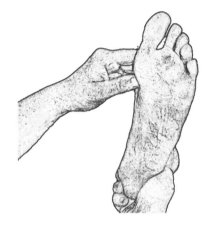 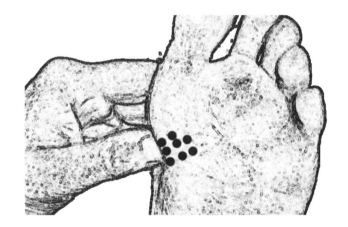

Helper reflexes- Adrenal- for the adrenaline.

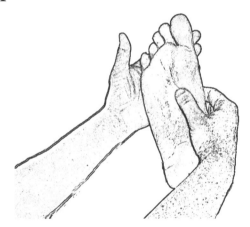 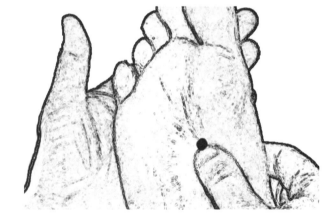

Chest & Lung- for the area of the heart.

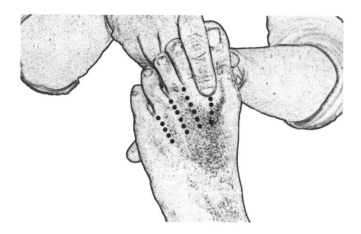 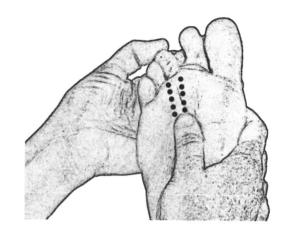

2nd Thoracic- the peripheral nerve that leads to the heart.

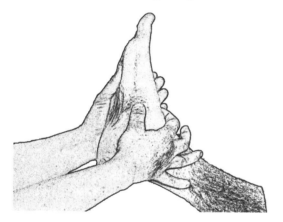 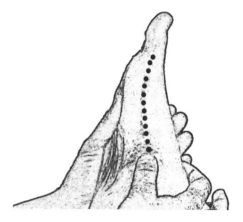

Parathyroid- to normalize muscle function.

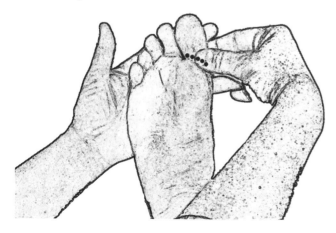 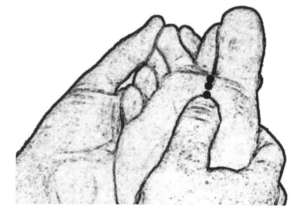

Diaphragm- to relieve tension near the heart area.

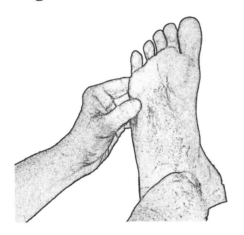 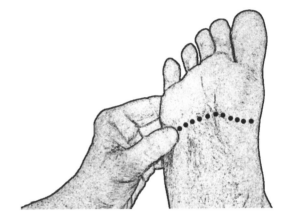

Sigmoid flexure- for build up of gas.

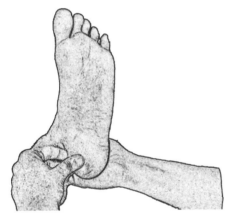 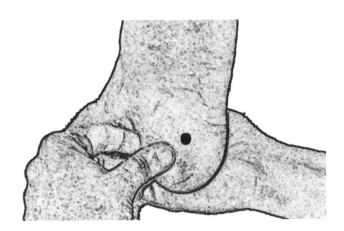

Atrial Fibrillation is an abnormal heart rhythm that occurs when the two small upper chambers of the heart, the atria, quiver instead of beating effectively. Blood is not pumped completely out of them when the heart beats, so it may pool and clot.

Direct Reflex- Heart

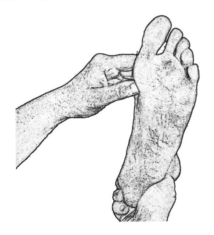 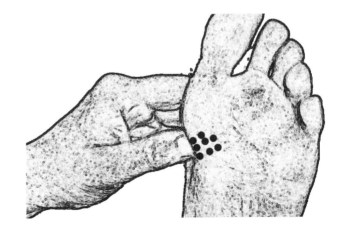

Helper Reflexes- Adrenal- for the adrenaline.

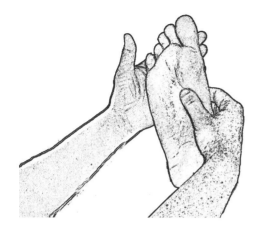
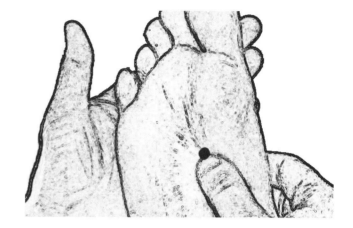

Chest & Lung- for the area of the heart.

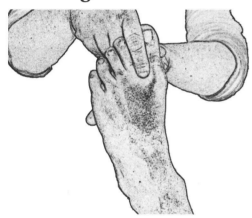
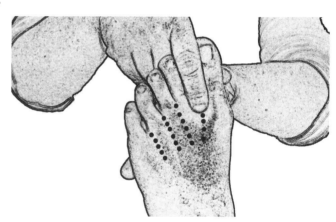

2nd Thoracic- the peripheral nerve that leads to the heart.

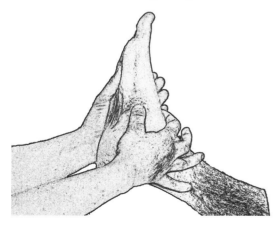
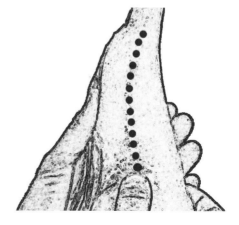

Parathyroid- to normalize muscle function.

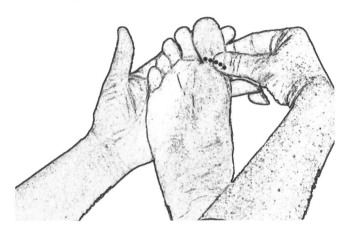 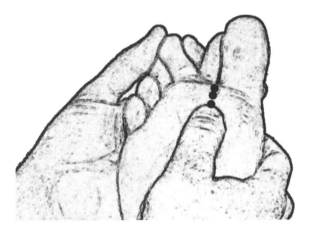

Diaphragm- to relieve tension in the heart area.

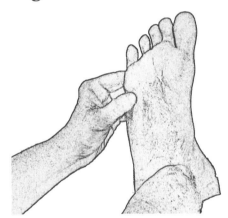 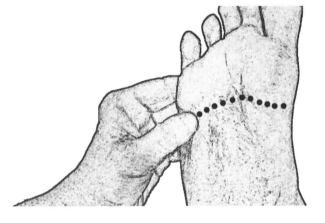

Sigmoid flexure- for a build up of gas.

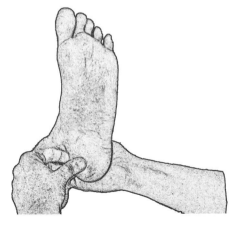 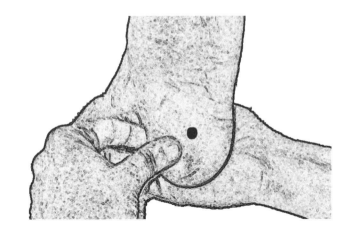

Heart Attack- is when one of the arteries supplying blood to the heart muscle becomes completely blocked by plaque and a blood clot at the site of narrowing.

Direct Reflexes- Heart

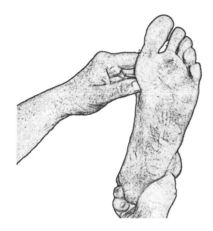 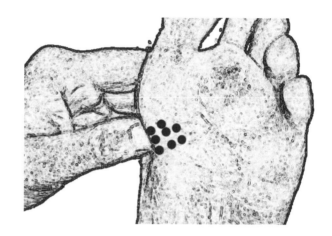

Helper Reflexes- Adrenal- for the adrenaline.

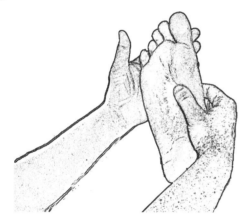 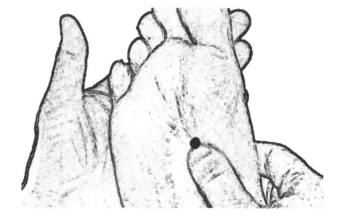

Chest & Lung- for the area of the heart.

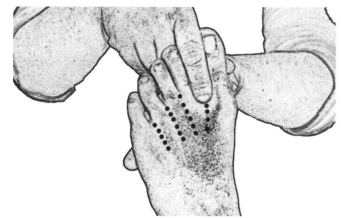 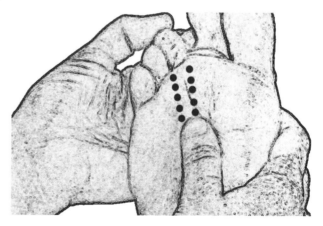

2nd Thoracic- for the peripheral nerve that leads to the heart.

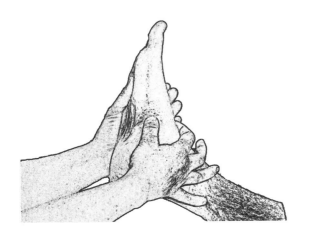 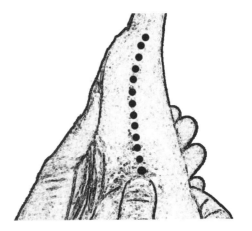

Parathyroid- to normalize muscle function.

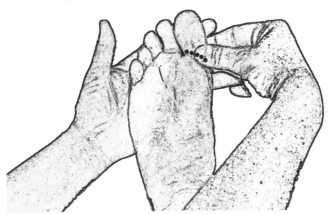 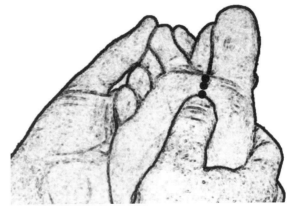

Diaphragm- to relieve tension.

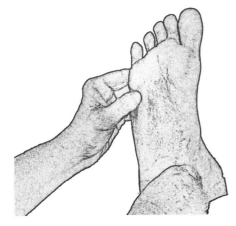 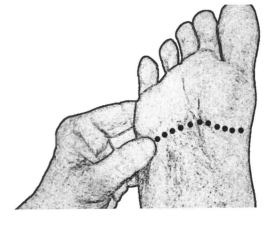

Sigmoid Flexure- for a build up of gas.

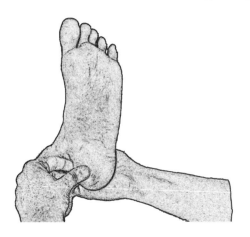
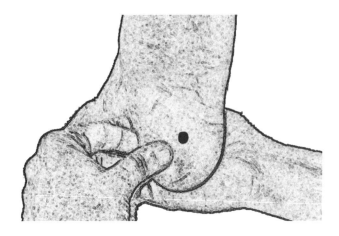

Pericarditis- is an inflammation of the pericardium, which is the thin sac membrane that surrounds the heart.

Direct Reflex- Heart

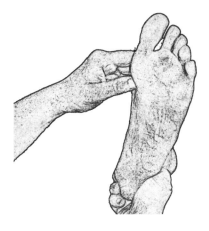
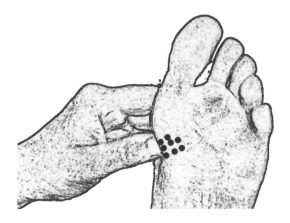

Helper Reflexes- Adrenal- for the inflammation.

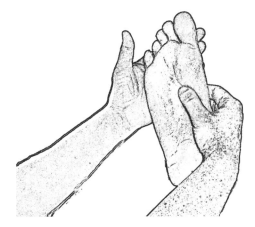
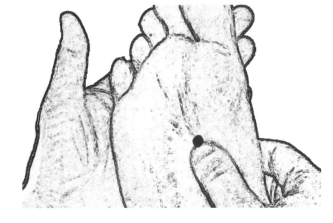

Chest & Lung- for the area of the heart.

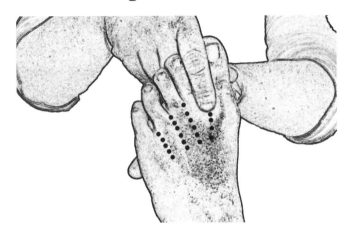 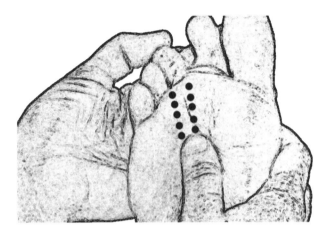

2nd & 9th Thoracic- for the peripheral nerve that leads to the heart and adrenal.

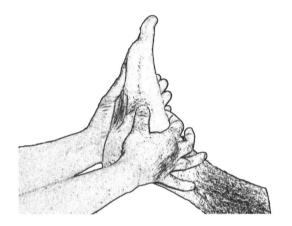 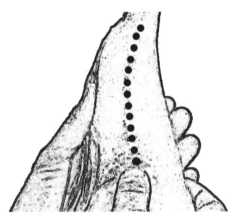

Quiz on the Circulatory System

1. How many sections is the heart divided?
   A) 2   B) 6   C)4

2. How many quarts of blood does the heart pump through the body?
   A) 7   B) 5   C) 9

3. Is the aorta the largest artery of the body?
   A) yes   B) no

4. Is the capillaries the smallest artery of the body?
   A) yes   B) no

5. Are veins the blood vessels that carry blood to the heart?
   A) yes   B) no

6. Where is the heart reflex located?
   A) plantar side on the waistline
   B) In Zones 4 & 5 on the diaphragm line
   C) In Zones 1 & 2 on the diaphragm line

* Answer key on page 325

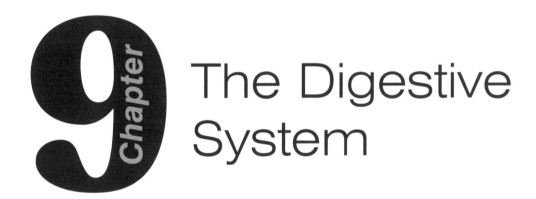

9

Chapter

The Digestive System

The Digestive System

The Digestive system is made up of hollow organs consisting of the mouth, pharynx, esophagus, stomach, small intestines, large intestines, rectum and anus. The outside of the digestive system consist of the liver, gallbladder, and the pancreas. The digestive system is responsible for digestion, absorption, and assimilation of fluids, vitamins, minerals, along with the elimination of wastes from the intestinal tract.

The Mouth is where digestion begins. The inner surface of the mouth is a mucous membrane. The salivary glands located in the cheeks and under the tongue secrete saliva. When the food is mixed with saliva the food reduces in size and this is the beginning of digestion process. The teeth are tools to break down the food. The tongue is used to taste and mix the food.
   The reflex areas are on the dorsal part of each foot about three-quarter inch down the great toe. Thumb-walk across this area.

The Pharynx is a muscular wall that helps to swallow food. It is connected to the esophagus to create a passageway for food to get to the stomach.
   The reflex areas are on plantar part of both feet on the great toe line. Thumb-walk across this area.

The Esophagus is a muscular tube that is about one foot long; It begins at the mouth and ends in the stomach.
   The reflex area is on the plantar part of the left foot, in Zone 1 on the ball of the foot. Thumb-walk starting from the diaphragm line to the toe line.

The Stomach is a storage area for food. It receives food via the esophagus. The stomach contracts, mixing food with enzymes (pepsin) and hydrochloric acid. (This is the beginning of digestion of proteins carries an limited amount of absorption moving food into the small intestines.)
   The reflex area is on the plantar part of the left foot under the diaphragm line in Zones 2, 3 and 4. Thumb-walk this area.

The Duodenum is where the stomach releases food into. It is the beginning of the small intestines. It is C shaped and 10 inches long. It receives pancreatic enzymes from the pancreas and bile from the liver. The food enters the duodenum through the pyloric sphincter in small amounts, so that the small intestines can digest.

The reflex area is on the plantar part of the right foot in Zone1 between the diaphragm line and the waistline. Thumb-walk this area.

The Small intestines is a twenty-two feet tubular organ located between the large intestine. It is a complex system of loops and coils which fills most of the abdomen. It receives secretions from the liver and the pancreas, finishes the digestion of the nutrients in chyme, absorbs products of digestion and removes the remaining to the large intestines.

The reflex areas are on the plantar part of both feet between the waist line and heel line in Zones 1-4. Thumb-walk this area.

The Ileocecal Valve is located between the small intestines and the large intestines. It prevents the back flow of fecal matter from the large to the small intestines, and also controls mucous secretion.

The reflex area is on the plantar part of the right foot in Zone 5 near the heel line. Thumb-press this area.

The Large intestines is a tube that is two inches in diameter and about five feet long. It absorbs electrolytes and forms and stores feces. It consist of four parts: the ascending, transverse, descending, and sigmoid. It plays only a small part of the digestion process.

The reflex areas are on the plantar part of both feet between the waistline and heel line in Zones 1-5. Thumb-walk the ascending in the fifth Zone, then across the waistline for the transverse on the right foot. On the left foot thumb-walk across the waistline for the transverse, then down Zone 5 for the descending and sigmoid.

The Sigmoid Flexure is an S-shaped section of the large colon. It is the last intestinal turn before the body wastes empty into the rectum for elimination. Gas is collected in this area.

The reflex area is on the plantar part of the left foot in Zone 4 past the heel line. Thumb-press this area.

The Liver is the largest organ and gland in the body. It is located on the right side under the rib cage. The liver has over 500 functions. The liver processes all the nutrients from the blood, storing fats, sugars, and proteins until the body needs them. It detoxifies the blood from alcohol and harmful chemicals. The liver manufactures bile, cholesterol, vitamin A, minerals, clotting factors, and complex proteins, while regulating the amount of glucose and protein entering the bloodstream for distribution to the body's tissue.

The reflex area is on the plantar part of the right foot under the diaphragm line in Zones 3,4, and 5. Thumb-walk this area.

The Gallbladder is nestled in the liver. It is a small sac linked by ducts to both liver and duodenum. It stores bile used for digestion by helping to counteract stomach acid and by aiding in the breaking down of fats. It also helps to lubricate the intestines.

The reflex area is on the plantar part of the right foot between the diaphragm line and waistline in Zone 4. Thumb-walk this area.

The Pancreas is located behind the lower part of the stomach and is about eight inches long, with its head attached to the duodenum and its tail extending up under the spleen. The large part of the pancreas manufactures digestive juices containing enzymes that flow down the pancreatic duct and into the duodenum, where it breaks down carbohydrates, fats and proteins into molecules that are small enough to be absorbed into the body. Scattered through the pancreas are tiny islands of cells--the Islets of Langerhans, which produce the hormones insulin and glucagon essential for metabolizing carbohydrates and regulating blood sugar.

The reflex areas are on the plantar part of both feet: on the right foot above the waistline in Zone 1. On the left foot above the waistline in Zones 1-4. Thumb-walk these areas.

Diagram of the Digestive System

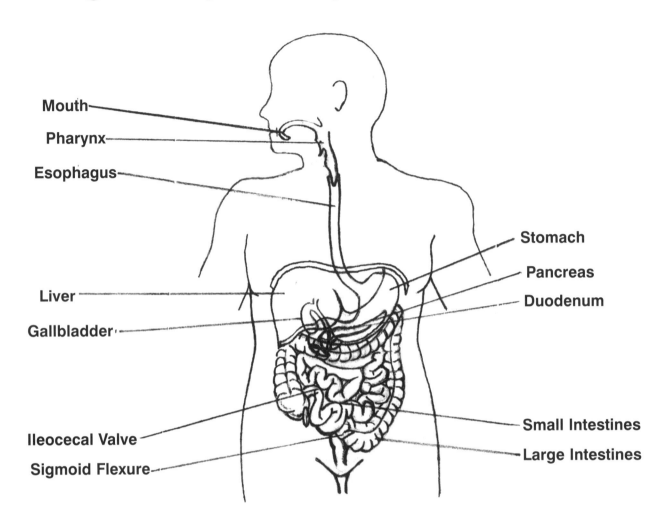

Locate the Reflex Areas of the Digestive System

*Use colored pencils and draw in the reflex areas

    A) Liver

    B) Gallbladder

    C) Stomach

    D) Esophagus

    E) Pancreas

    F) Duodenum

    G) Small intestines

    H) Ileocecal valve

    I) Ascending colon

    J) Transverse colon

    K) Descending colon

    L) Sigmoid flexure

    M) Rectum / hemorrhoids

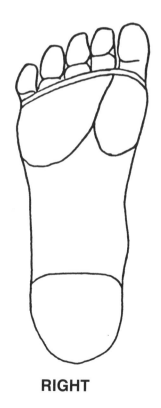

RIGHT

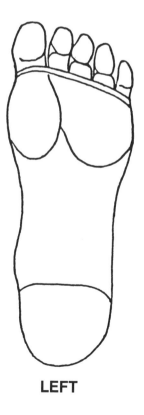

LEFT

*Answer key on next page

Answer Key to the Digestive Reflex Areas

Stomach

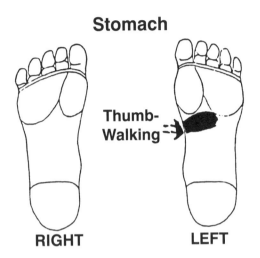

Thumb-Walking

RIGHT LEFT

Liver/Gallbladder

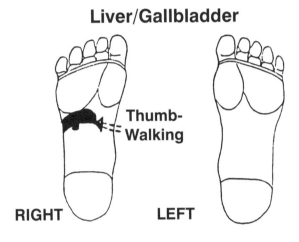

Thumb-Walking

RIGHT LEFT

Pancreas

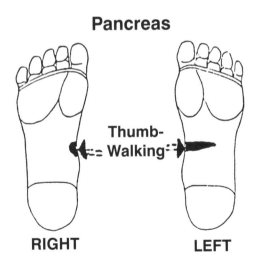

Thumb-Walking

RIGHT LEFT

Large Intestine

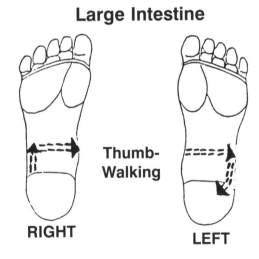

Thumb-Walking

RIGHT LEFT

Answer Key to the Digestive Reflex Areas

Small Intestines

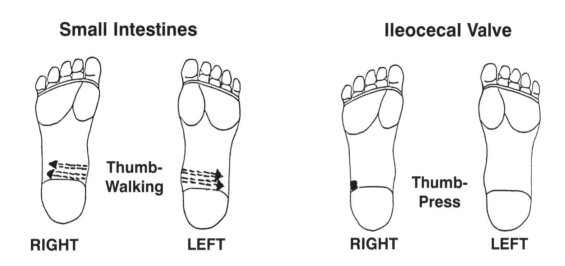

Ileocecal Valve

Sigmoid Flexure

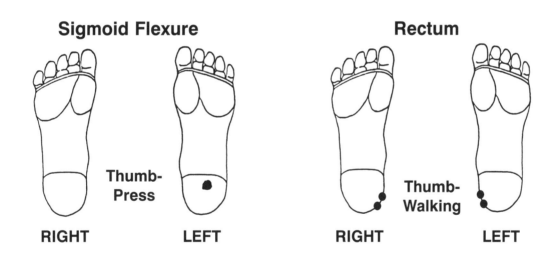

Rectum

How to Work the Digestive Reflex Areas

The **Esophagus reflex area** is on the left foot on the plantar (bottom) part, in Zone 1, starting from the diaphragm line up towards the toes. Thumb-walk this area.

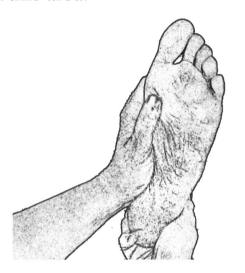
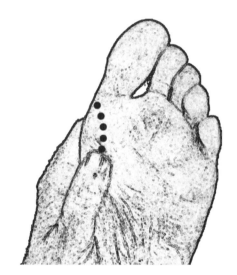

The **Duodenum reflex area** is on the right foot on the plantar (bottom) part, in Zone 1, starting from the waistline on the medial (inside) of the foot. Thumb-walk up this area.

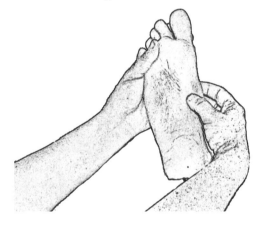
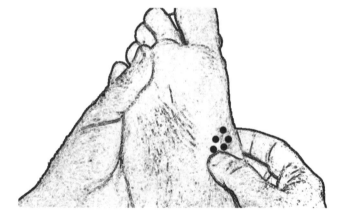

The **Small Intestines reflex areas** are on both feet on the plantar (bottom) part, in Zones 1-4. Thumb-walk these areas.

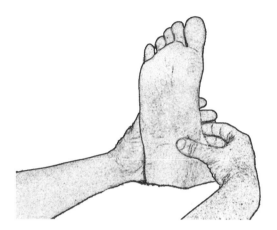
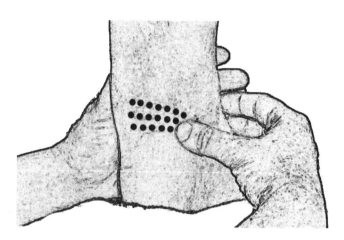

The **Ileocecal Valve reflex area** is on the right foot on the plantar (bottom) part, in Zone 5, at the heel line. Thumb-press this area.

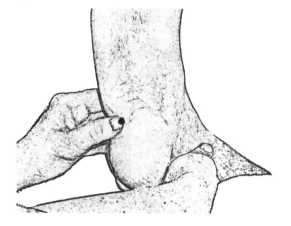
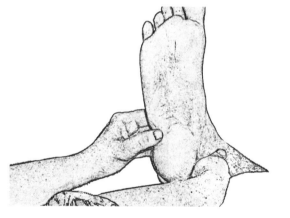

The **Ascending Colon reflex area** is on the right foot, on the plantar (bottom) part, in Zone 5. Thumb-walk up this area.

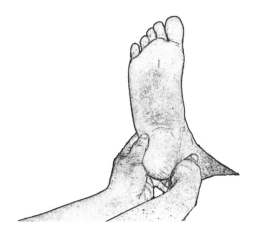
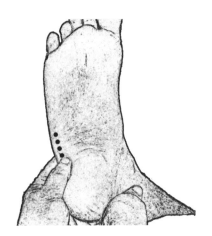

The **Transverse Colon reflex areas** are on both feet, on the plantar (bottom) part, in Zones 1-5, below the waistline.

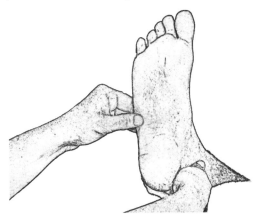
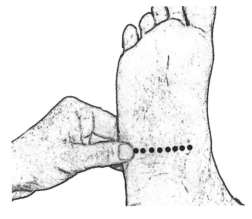

The **Descending Colon reflex area** is on the left foot, plantar (bottom) part, in Zone 5, starting at the waistline to the heel line. Thumb-walk down this area.

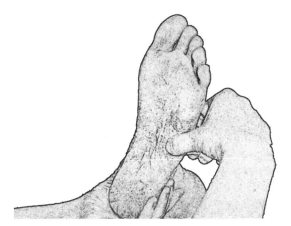 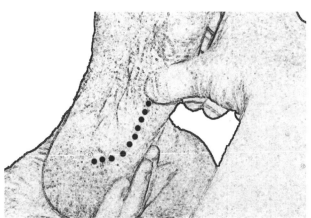

The **Sigmoid Flexure reflex area** is on the left foot, plantar (bottom) part, between Zones 3-4, past the heel line. Thumb-press this area.

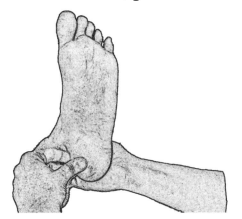 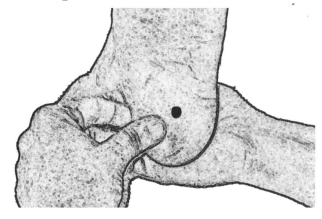

The **Liver and Gallbladder reflex area** is on the right foot, on the plantar (bottom) part, in Zones 2-4, starting from two inches above the waistline to the diaphragm line. Thumb-walk this area.

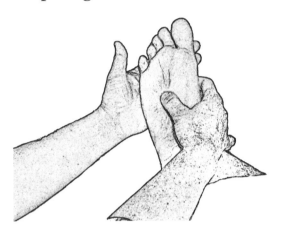
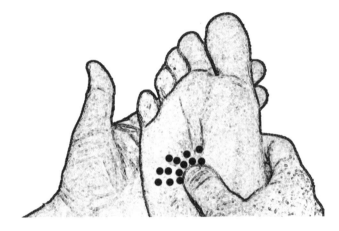

The **Stomach reflex area** is on the left foot, on the plantar (bottom) part, in Zones 2-4, starting from two inches above the waistline to the diaphragm line. Thumb-walk this area.

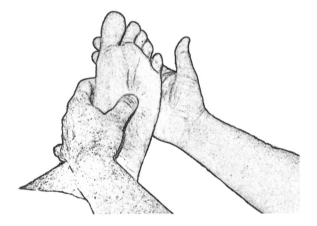
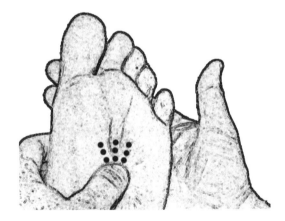

The **Pancreas reflex areas** are on both feet, on the plantar (bottom) part. On the right foot, it is in Zone 1, above the waistline; on the left foot it is in Zones 1-4, above the waistline. Thumb-walk these areas.

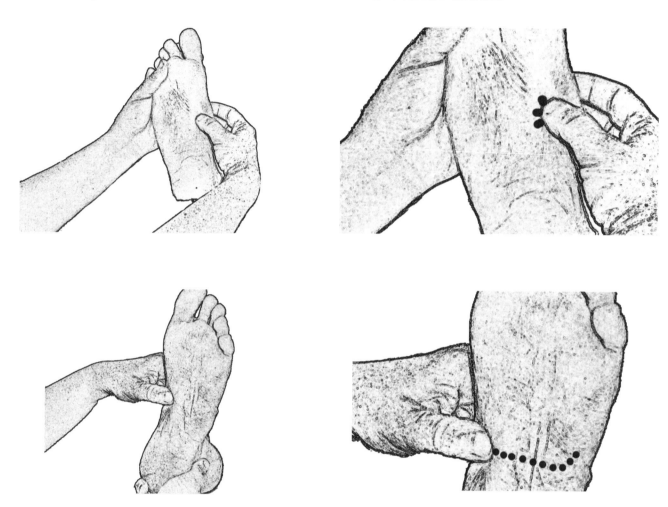

Digestive Disorders and the Helper Reflex Areas

Constipation- difficulty passing hard bowel movements.

Direct Reflex-

Large colon for controlling water in the colon

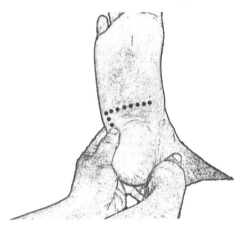
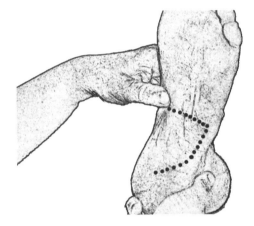

Sigmoid flexure for gas pain.

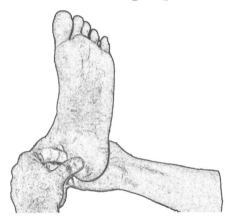
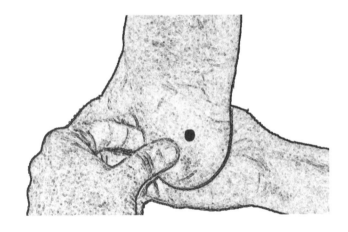

Helper Reflexes- Adrenal to tone the muscles.

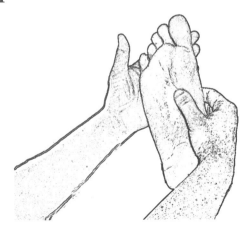
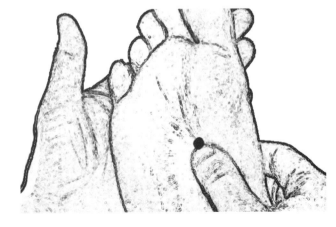

Gallbladder/Liver it lubricates the colon.

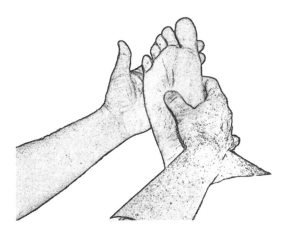 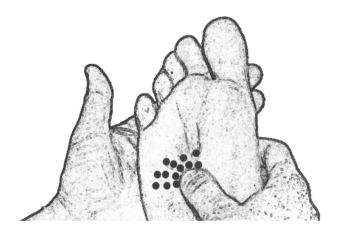

Ileocecal valve to release mucous for lubrication.

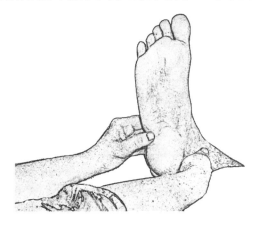 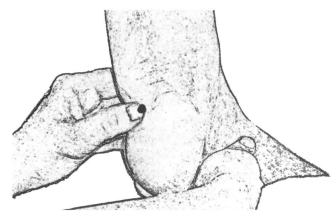

Lumbar/Coccyx this peripheral nerve leads to the colon.

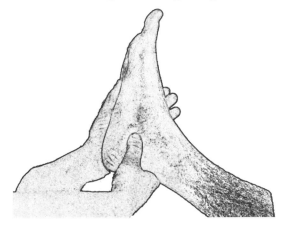 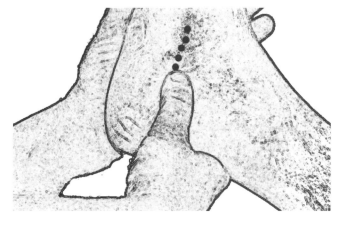

Solar plexus helps with relaxation.

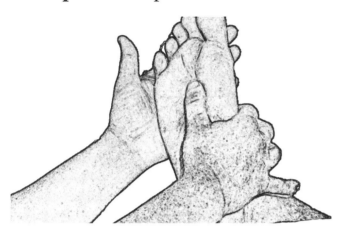
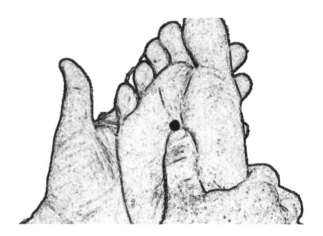

Crohn's disease is a chronic inflammation of the final section of the small intestines.

Direct Reflex- Small intestines to help control loose bowels.

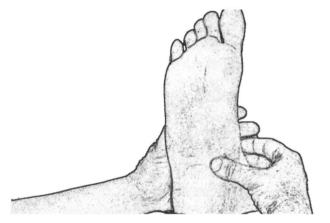
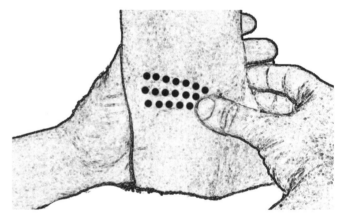

Helper Reflexes- Adrenal for inflammation.

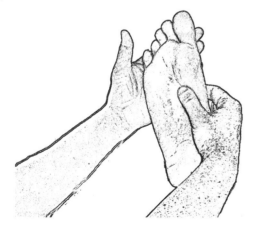
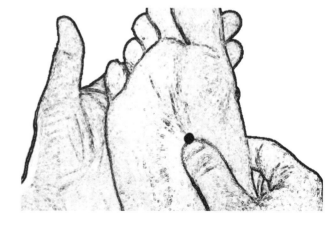

Duodenum for blood supply.

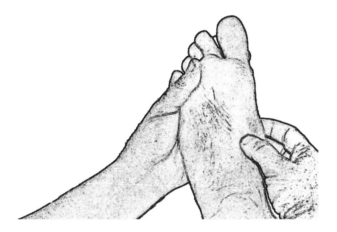 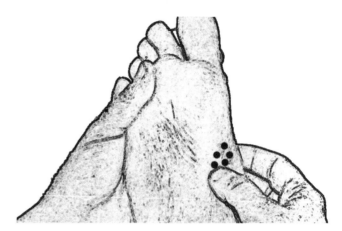

Ileocecal valve for controlling mucous.

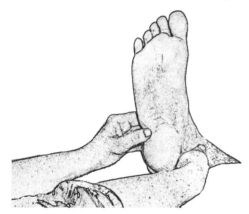 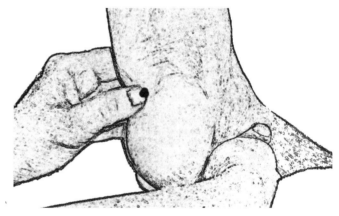

Gallbladder/Liver to control bile.

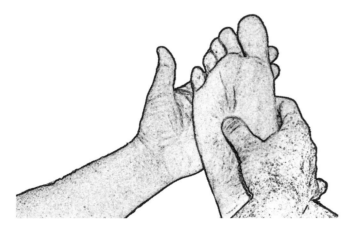 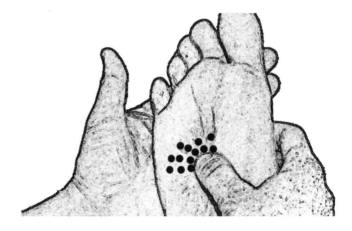

Thoracic for nerve supply.

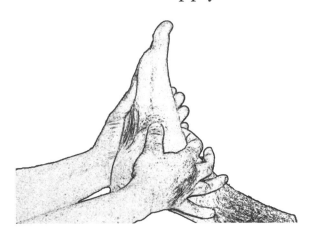 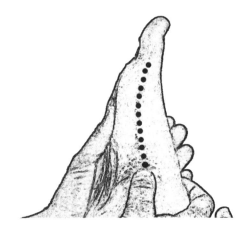

Lumbar for nerve supply.

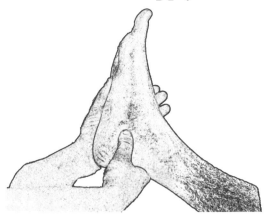 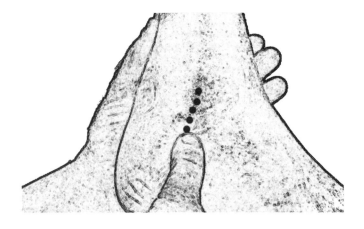

Solar Plexus for stress and tension.

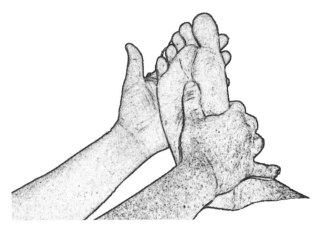 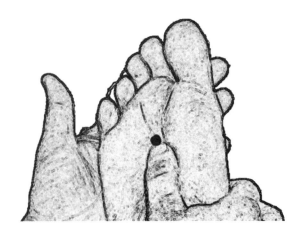

Diarrhea- loose watery bowels.

Direct Reflex- Small intestines to control loose bowels.

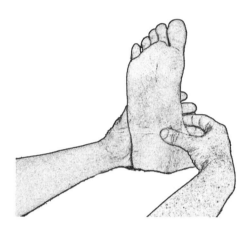 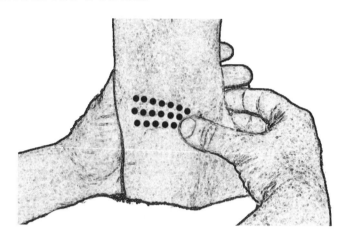

Helper Reflexes- Adrenal to balance the amount of water and to tone the muscle.

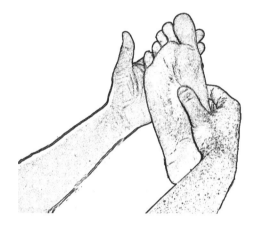 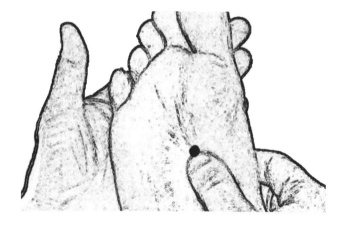

Duodenum for blood supply.

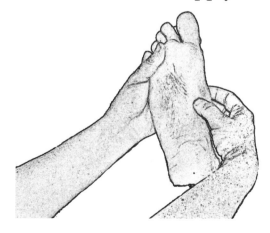 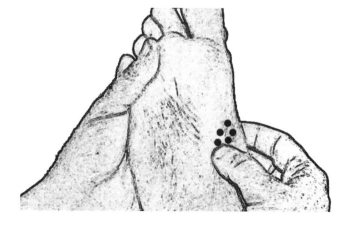

Thoracic for nerve supply.

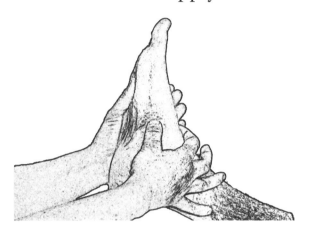
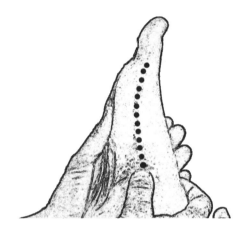

Lumbar for nerve supply.

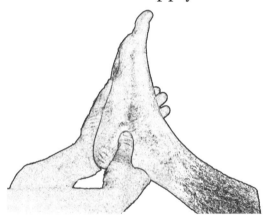
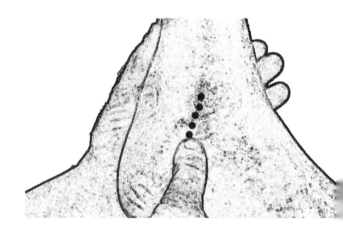

Solar Plexus for stress and tension.

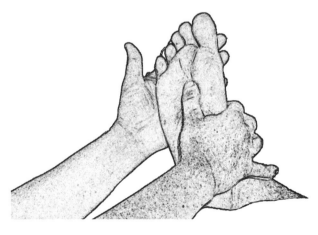
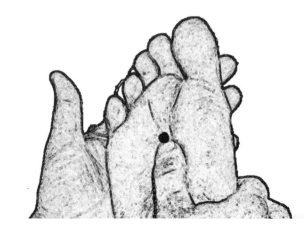

Large colon for controlling water in the colon.

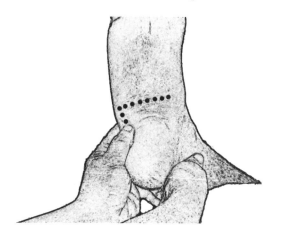
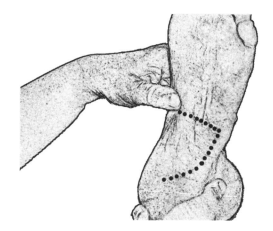

Gallbladder/Liver for controlling the bile.

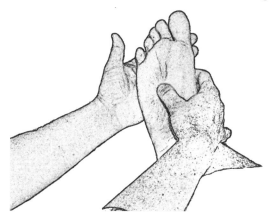
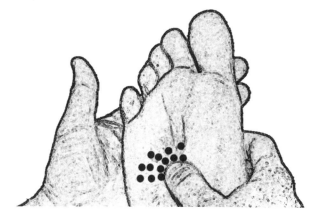

Thoracic for nerve supply.

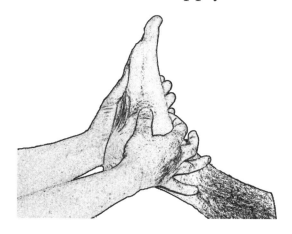
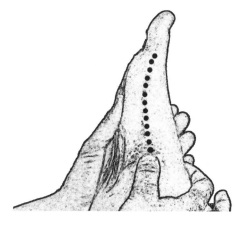

Lumbar for nerve supply.

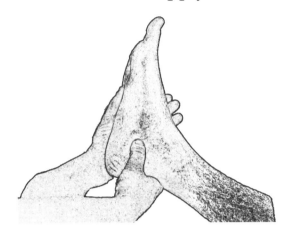
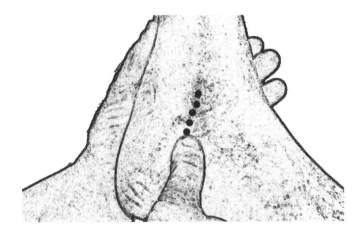

Solar plexus to relax.

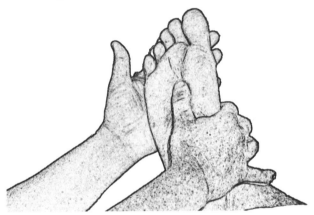
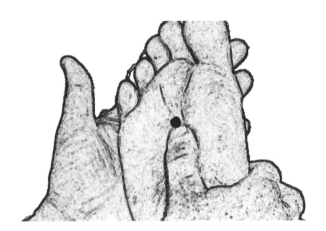

Diabetes- the amount of glucose in the blood is controlled by the hormones insulin and glucagon; Too much can cause the blood sugar to rise too high. Type 1- a disease in which the body does not produce insulin, occurring in children. Type 2- a disorder caused by the body's inability to make enough insulin.

Direct Reflex- Pancreas to control blood sugar.

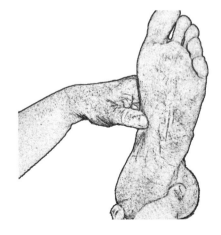
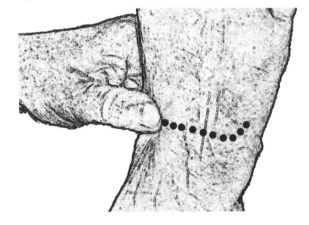

Helper Reflexes- Adrenal to control the body's carbohydrate use.

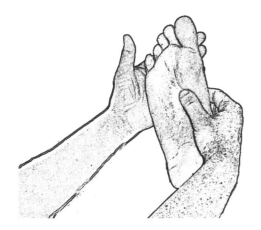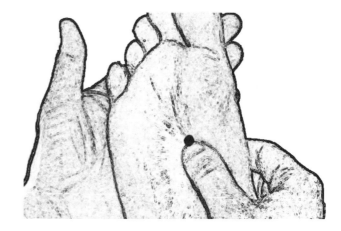

Liver stores sugar until it needs it.

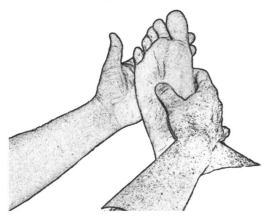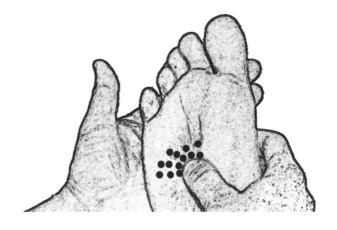

Pituitary regulates sugar content in the blood.

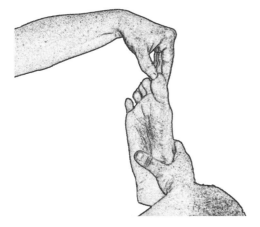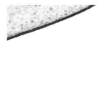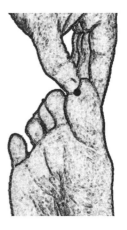

7th Thoracic for nerve supply to the pancreas.

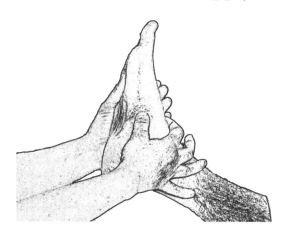
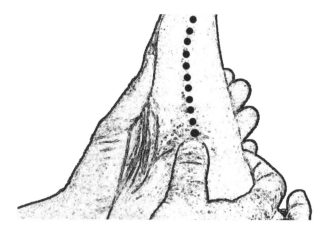

Diverticulosis- is a small sac-like swelling that develop in the walls of the lower colon. When the sac becomes inflamed the condition is called diverticulitis.

Direct Reflex- Descending colon

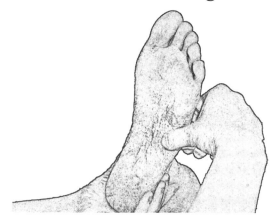
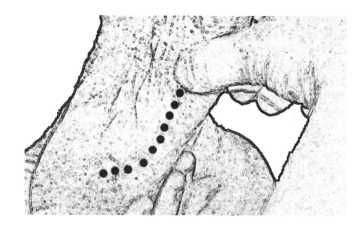

Sigmoid flexure for gas pain.

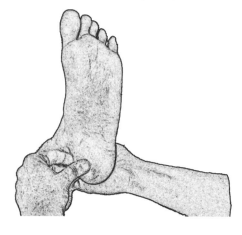
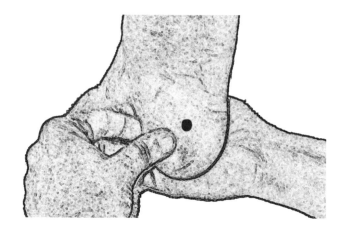

Helper Reflexes- **Adrenal** for inflammation.

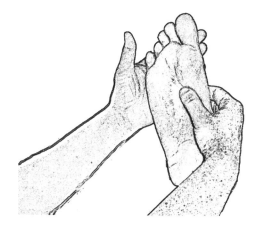
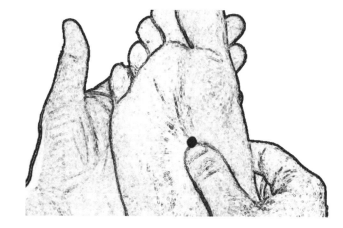

Gallbladder/Liver to lubricate.

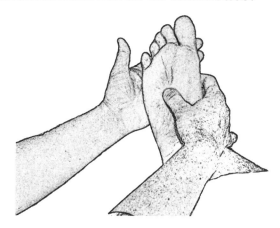
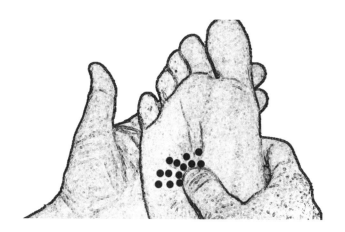

Lumbar/Sacral for nerve supply.

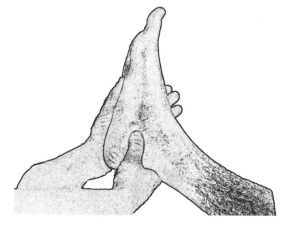
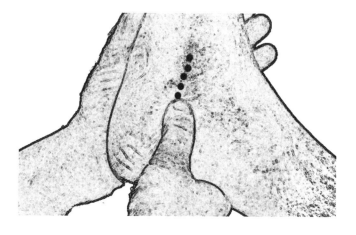

Solar Plexus to relax.

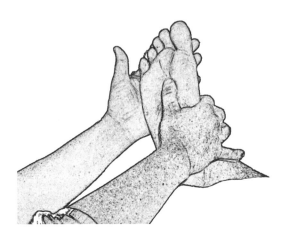
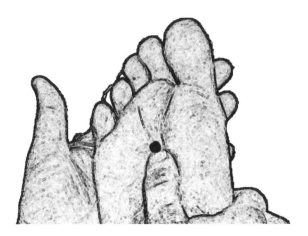

Gallstones- are stone-like fatty cholesterol substances that form in the gallbladder.

Direct Reflex- Gallbladder to break down the fats.

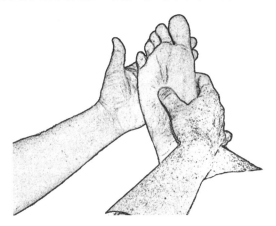
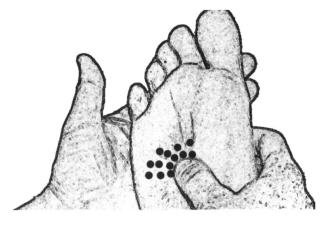

Helper Reflexes- Liver controls cholesterol levels.

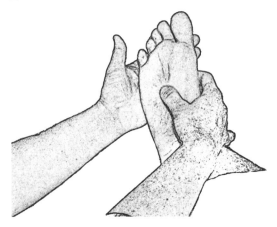
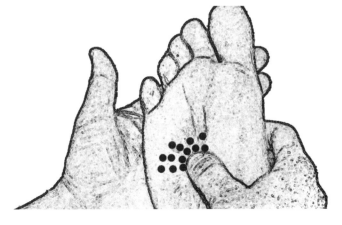

Parathyroid controls calcium levels.

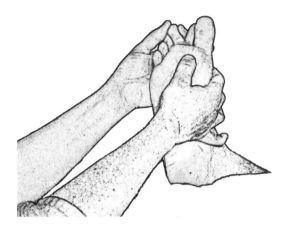 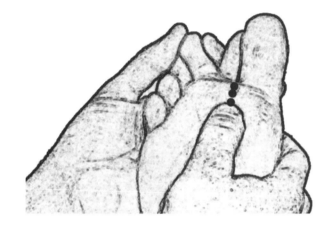

Thyroid controls cholesterol levels.

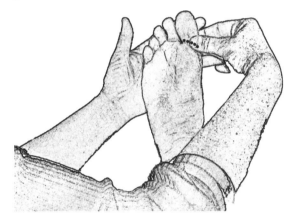 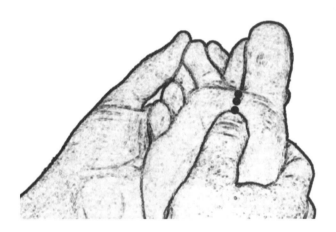

Heartburn/Reflux disease- the stomach acidic juices travel back up the esophagus, because of a digestive disorder that affects the lower esophageal sphincter (the muscle connecting the esophagus with the stomach.)

Direct Reflex- Esophagus aids better blood supply.

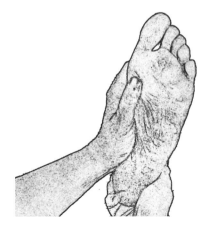 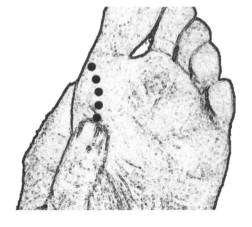

Stomach helps to release pepsin.

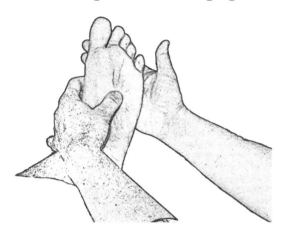
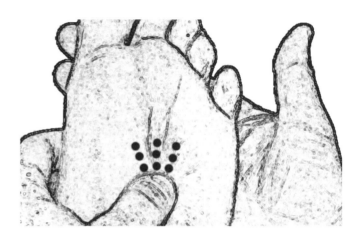

Helper Reflexes- Gallbladder/Liver controls bile and helps to digest fats.

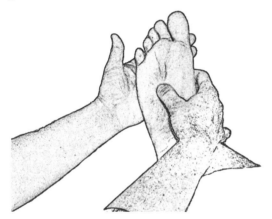
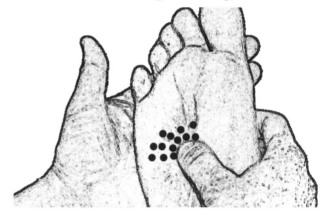

Solar plexus to relax.

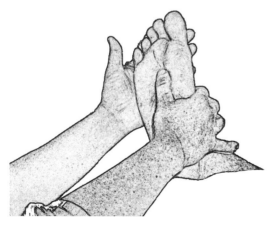
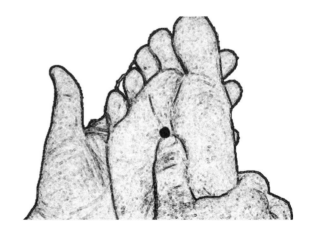

Hemorrhoids- are like varicose veins on either side of the anus.

Direct Reflex- Rectum/ hemorrhoids.

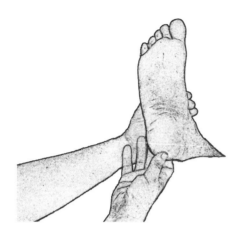
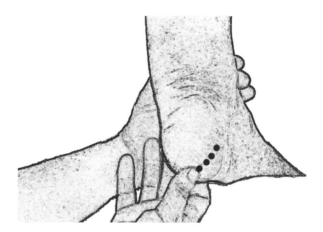

Helper Reflexes- Adrenal helps for inflammation.

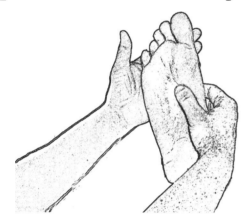
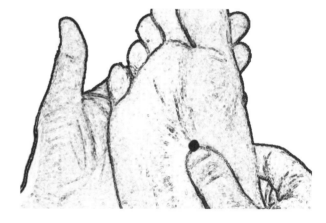

Sigmoid flexure helps for elimination.

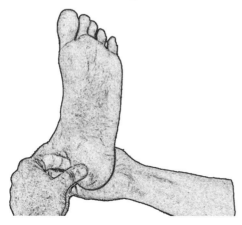
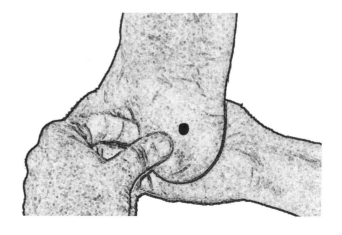

Hypoglycemia- is the amount of glucose in the blood and is controlled by the hormones insulin and glucagon. Too little can cause blood sugar to fall too low.

Direct Reflex- Pancreas to help regulate blood sugar.

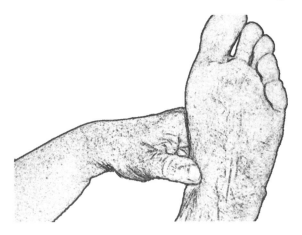 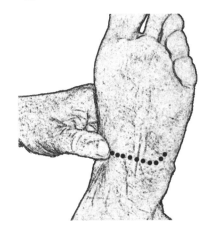

Helper Reflexes- Adrenal helps to control fats and carbohydrates.

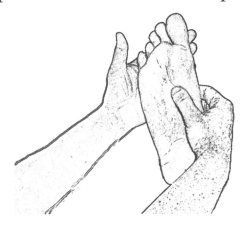 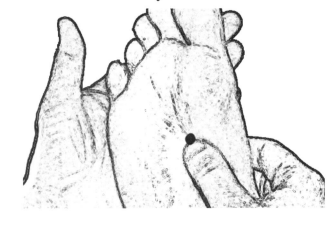

Liver it stores sugar.

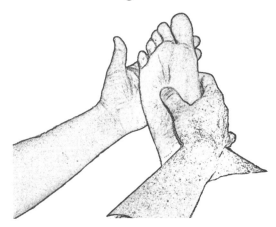 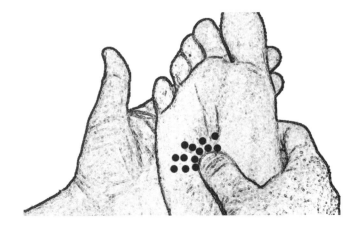

Pituitary it controls sugar content in the blood.

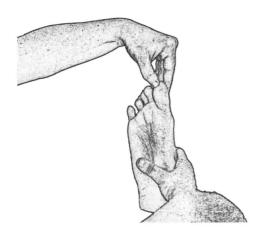 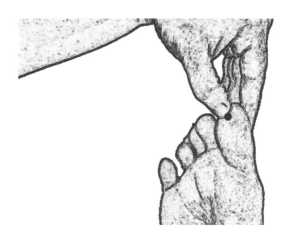

Irritable Bowel Syndrome- is a common disorder of the intestines that leads to cramping, gassiness, and bloating. Some people have constipation, while others have diarrhea.

Direct Reflex- Large colon it helps to normalize and create better water balance.

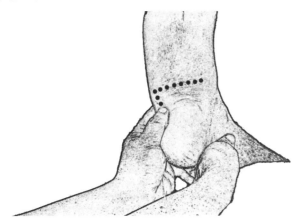 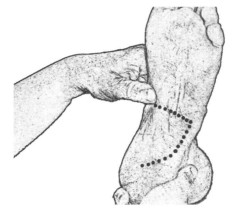

Helper Reflexes- Ileocecal valve it controls mucous secretions.

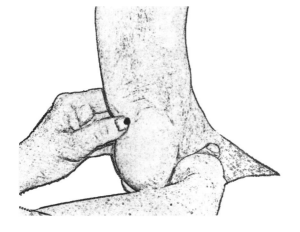 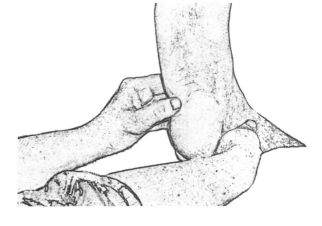

Sigmoid flexure it helps for elimination.

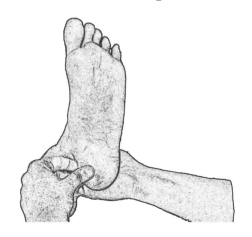
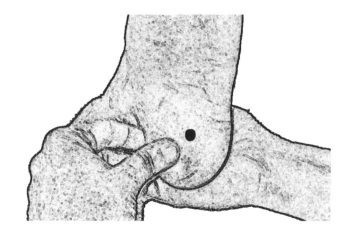

Small intestines helps the remaining nutrients into the large intestines.

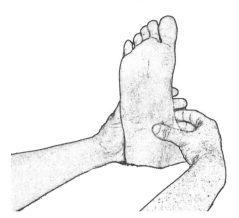
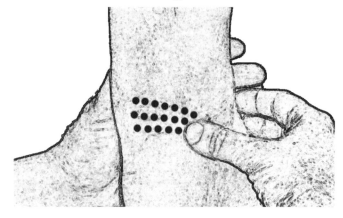

Gallbladder/Liver helps to release digestive juices.

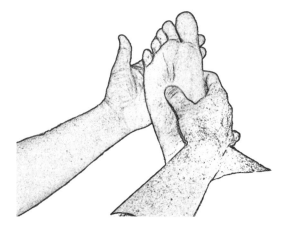
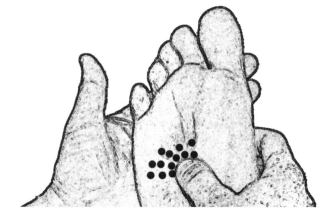

Lumbar the peripheral nerve leads to the colon.

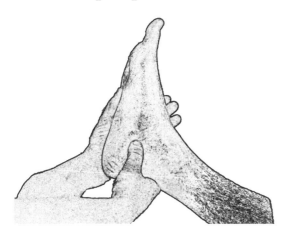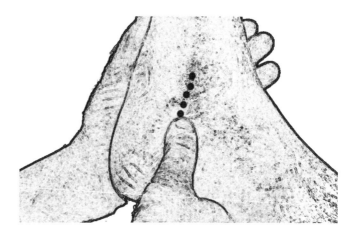

Morning sickness- nausea during the first four months of pregnancy.

Direct Reflex- Stomach to help release digestive juices.

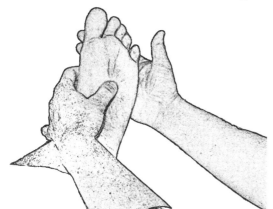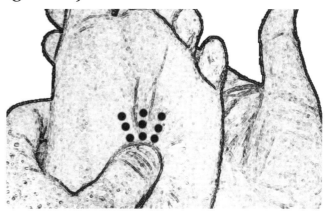

Helper reflexes- All glands helps to regulate the body.

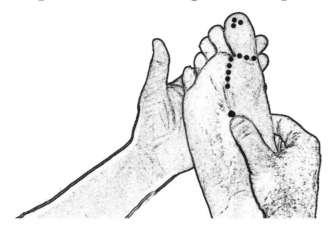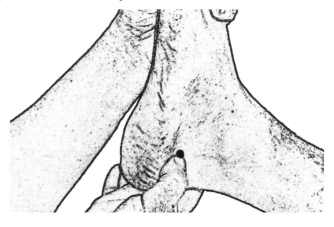

Solar plexus helps to relax.

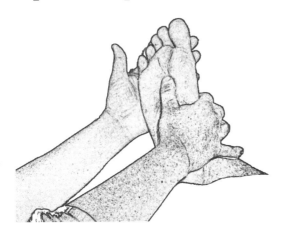
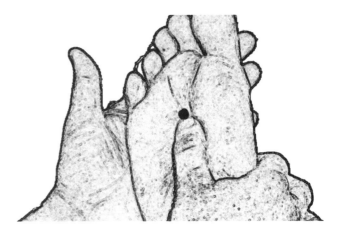

Motion sickness- nausea caused by motion from a vehicle, airplane, or boat.

Direct Reflex- Ears to balance.

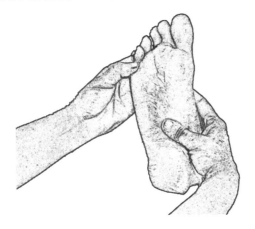
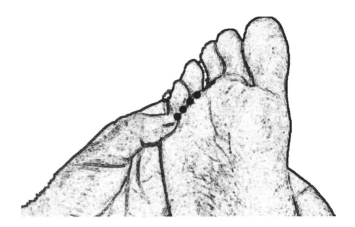

Helper Reflexes- All neck reflexes to help with blood supply.

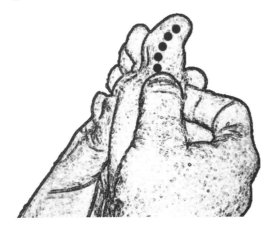
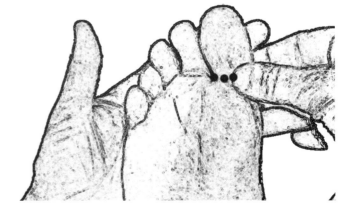

Stomach for nausea.

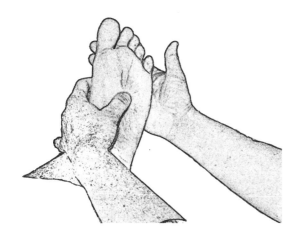
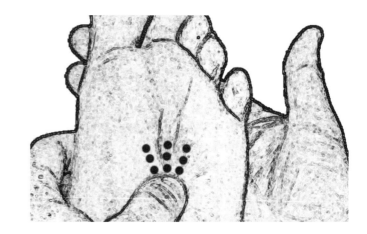

Solar plexus to relax.

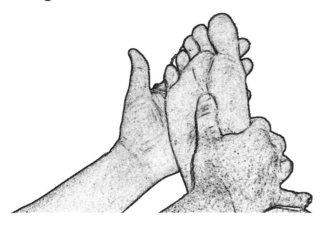
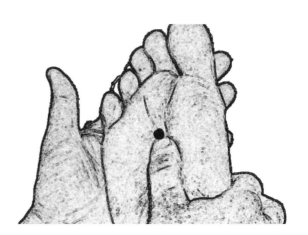

Nausea- a stomach upset that may cause vomiting.

Direct Reflex - Stomach for nausea.

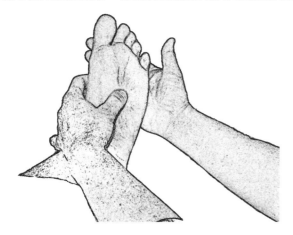
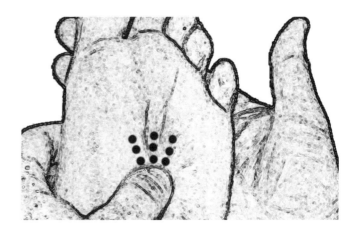

Helper Reflexes- Gallbladder/Liver to help digest.

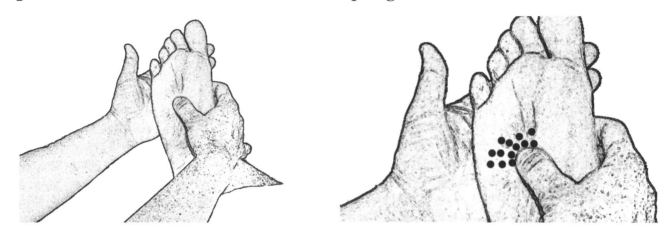

Solar plexus to help relax stress and tension.

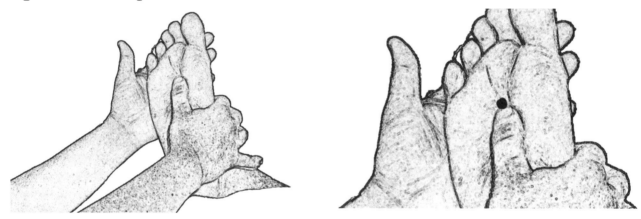

Ulcer- is a sore on the stomach or duodenum lining. It could be caused by stress or a bacterial infection.

Direct Reflex- Duodenum to aid better blood supply to heal the sore.

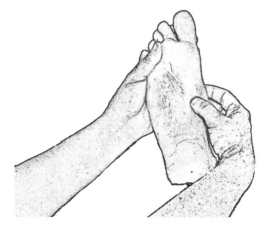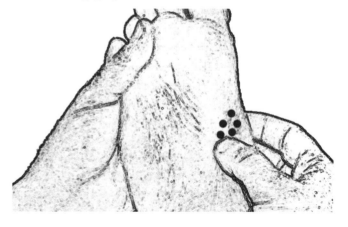

Stomach to aid better blood supply to heal the stomach.

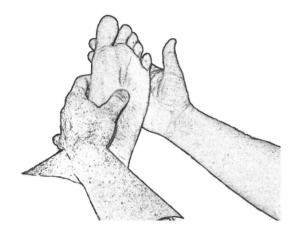 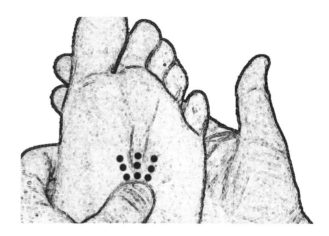

Helper Reflexes- Adrenal to help with stress and tension.

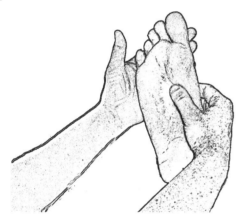 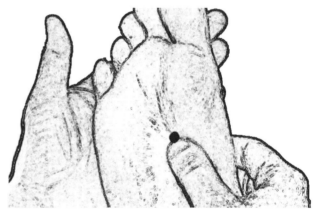

Solar plexus to help with stress and tension.

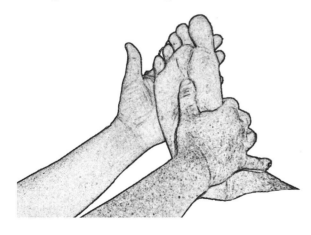 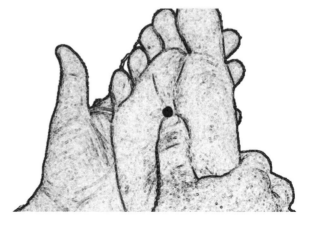

Quiz on the Digestive System

1. The pharynx does what job in the digestive system?
   A) muscular wall to help swallow food
   B) storage area for food
   C) muscular tube that begins at the mouth and ends in the stomach

2. The ileocecal valve does what in the digestive system?
   A) controls mucous secretion
   B) receives secretions from the liver and pancreas
   C) releases food into the duodenum

3. Where is the ileocecal valve reflex area located?
   A) Zone 1 at the heel line   B) Zone 5 at the heel line
   C) Zone 3 above the heel line

4. The liver does what job in the digestive system?
   A) stores bile   B) manufactures digestive juices containing enzymes
   C) manufactures vitamins and minerals

5. Where is the liver reflex located?
   A) left foot only under the diaphragm line in Zones 2 and 3
   B) right foot only under the diaphragm line in Zones 3, 4, and 5
   C) Both feet under the diaphragm line in Zones 2, 3, and 4

6. The stomach does what job in the digestive system
   A) mixes food with enzymes and hydrochloric acids
   B) manufactures digestive juices containing enzymes   C) stores bile

7. Where is the stomach reflex area located?
   A) right foot only   B) left foot only   C) both feet

8. The pancreas does what job in the digestive system?
   A) breaks down carbohydrates, fats, and proteins
   B) manufactures vitamins and minerals   C) stores bile

9. Where is the pancreas reflex area located?
   A) both feet on the waistline B) right foot only at the waistline
   C) left foot only on the waistline

* Answer key on page 325

10

Urinary System

Urinary System

The Urinary System consist of the kidneys, ureter tube, bladder, and urethra. The urinary system keeps the chemicals and water in balance by removing waste called urea from the blood. Urea is produced when protein from meat products are broken down in the body.

The Kidneys are located about two inches above the body's mid-line just below and behind the liver and lower ribs. They remove and purify many pints of blood per hour and circulated to the rest of the body. The kidneys regulate retention of important minerals and water. The kidneys are the master filters of the body.

The kidney reflex areas are found on the plantar (bottom) part on both feet between Zones 2 and 3 just above the waistline. Thumb-walk this area.

The Bladder is a hollow triangle shaped muscular organ in the lower abdomen that stores urine. The adult bladder can hold up to a pint of fluid. It is suspended by ligaments that attach to other organs and to the pelvic bone.

The bladder reflex areas are found on the plantar (bottom) medial (inside) part on both feet just above the heel line, in Zone 1. Thumb-walk this area.

The Ureter Tubes these are two uterine tubes that carry urine from the kidney to the bladder. Each ureter is ten to twelve inches long. Urine flows down partially by gravity, but mainly by waves of contractions through the muscular layers of the urethral walls.

The ureter tube reflex areas are found on the plantar (bottom) part on both feet starting above the heel line, in Zone 1 from the bladder thumb-walk to the kidney reflex in Zones 2 and 3.

Urethra is a tube that connects from the bladder to the outside of the body. It is a wall that is lined with mucous membranes and it has a thick layer of smooth muscle tissue. It contains many mucous glands that secretes mucous in to the urethral canal.

The urethra reflex areas are found on the plantar (bottom) medial (inside) part on both feet at the heel line, in Zone 1. Thumb-walk this area.

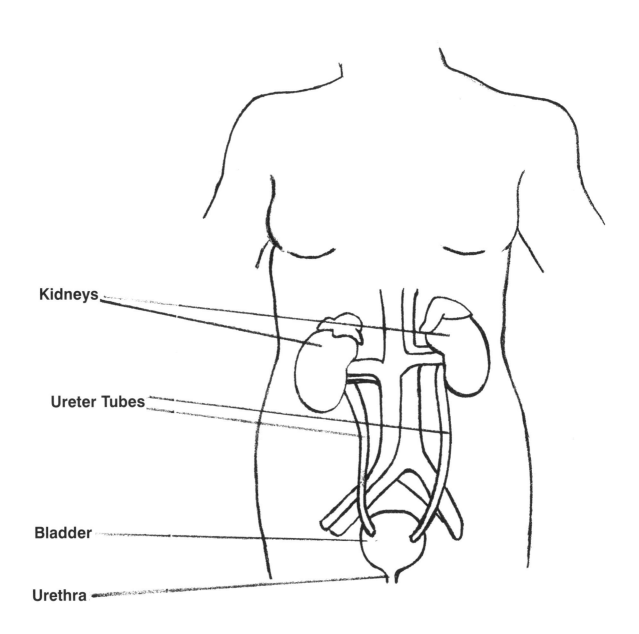

Locate the Reflex areas of the Urinary System

*Use colored pencils to draw in reflex areas

    A) Bladder

    B) Ureter Tube

    C) Kidney

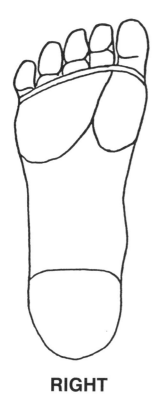 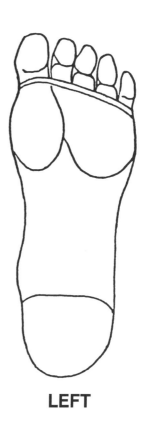

RIGHT   **LEFT**

*Answer key on next page

Answer Key to the Urinary Reflex Areas

Kidneys

Ureter Tubes

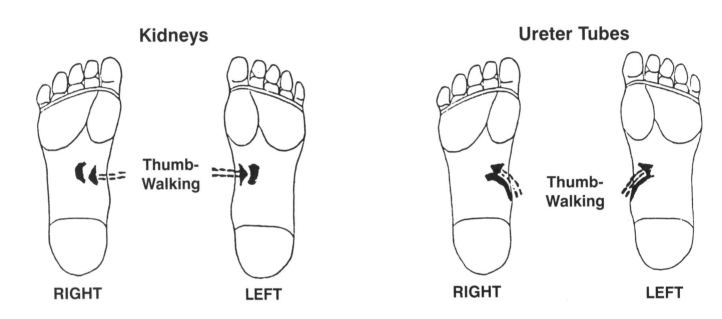

RIGHT   Thumb-Walking   LEFT

RIGHT   Thumb-Walking   LEFT

Bladder

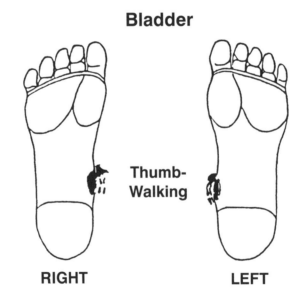

RIGHT   Thumb-Walking   LEFT

How to Work the Urinary System Reflex Areas

The **Bladder reflex areas** are on both feet in Zone 1 on the medial side, about one inch from the heel line. Thumb-walk these areas.

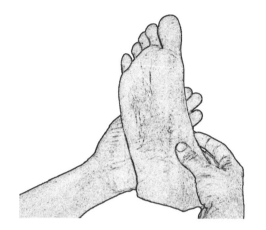
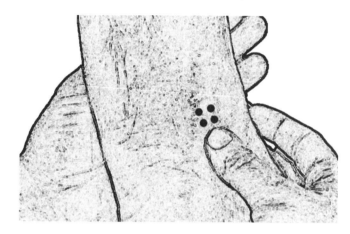

The **Ureter Tube reflex areas** are on both feet in Zones 1-2. Thumb-walk from the bladder to the kidney reflex.

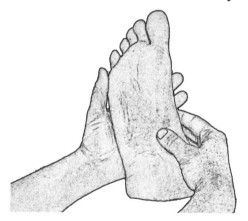
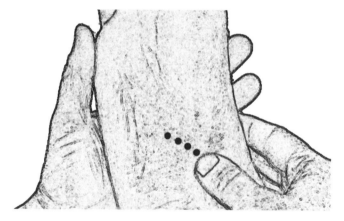

The **Kidney reflex areas** are on both feet in Zones 2-3 on the waistline. Thumb-walk these areas.

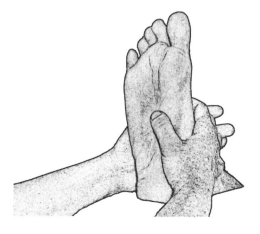
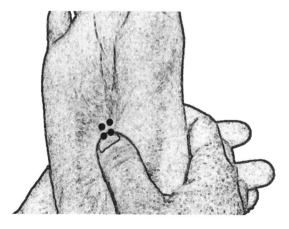

Urinary Disorders and the Helper Reflex Areas

Bed-wetting

Direct Reflex- the complete Urinary System, to strengthen.

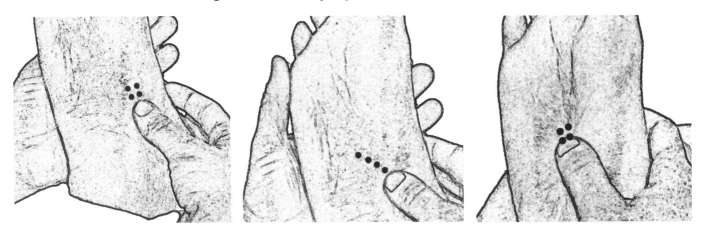

Helper Reflexes- Adrenal to tone the muscle.

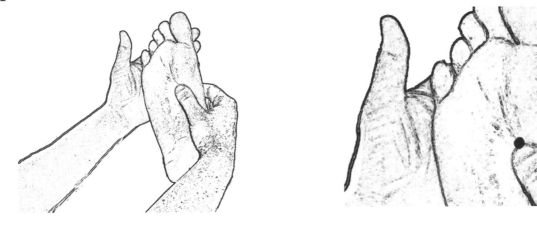

3rd Lumbar the peripheral nerve that leads to the kidney.

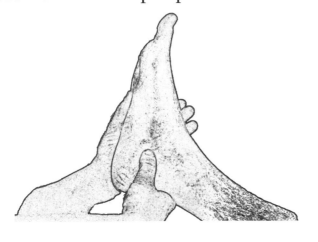
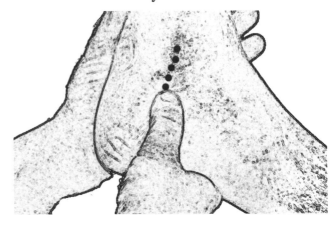

Diaphragm to help relax.

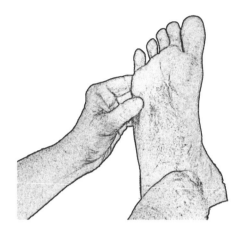
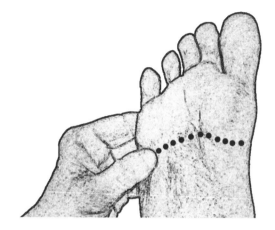

Cystitis- is a chronic inflammatory condition of the bladder. The protective layers of the bladders interior surface breaks down, allowing the toxins from the urine to irritate the bladder wall and causes inflammation.

Direct Reflex- Bladder

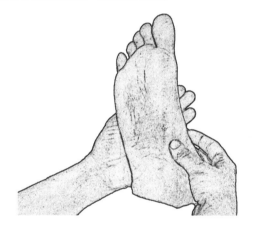
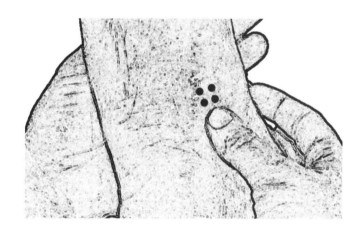

Helper Reflexes- Adrenal for inflammation and for muscle tone.

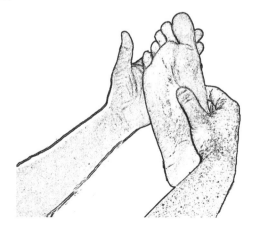
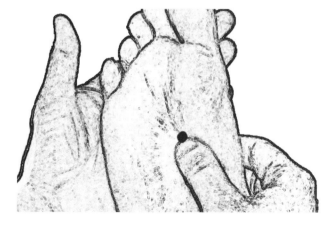

3rd Lumbar for nerve supply.

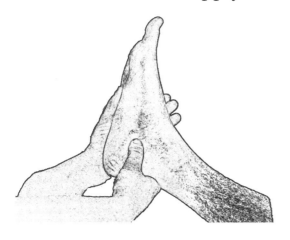 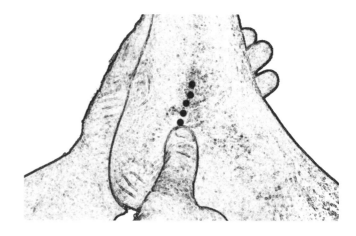

Kidneys to strengthen.

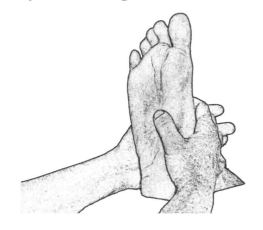 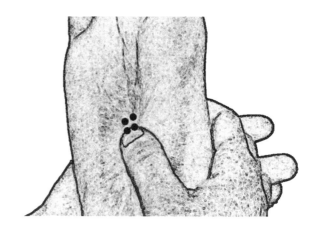

Incontinence- is the inability to hold urine.

Direct Reflex- Bladder

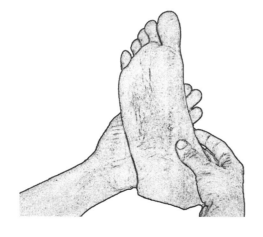 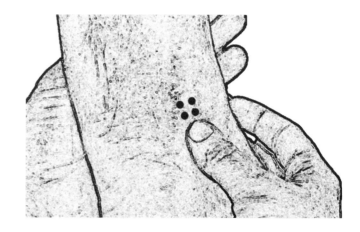

Helper Reflexes- Adrenal for toning the muscles.

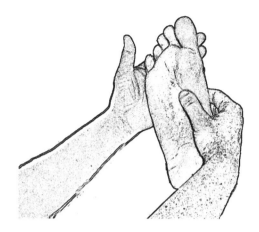 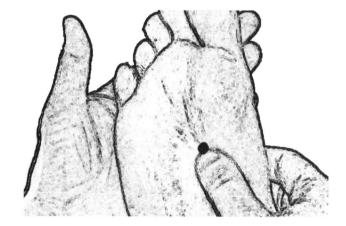

Kidneys for better blood supply.

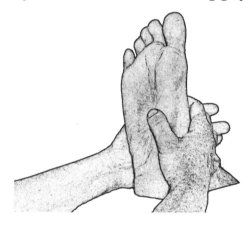 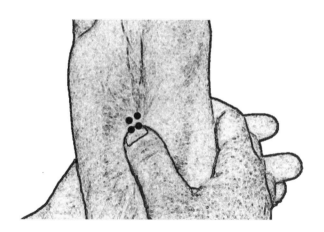

Ureter Tube to strengthen the muscular wall.

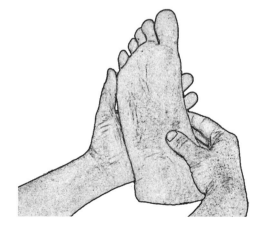 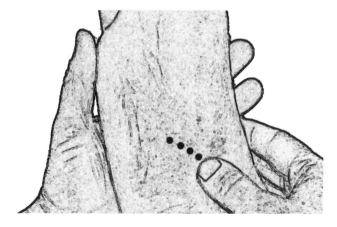

10th and 11th Thoracic for nerve supply to kidneys and ureters.

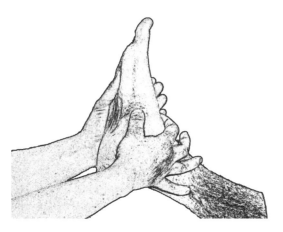 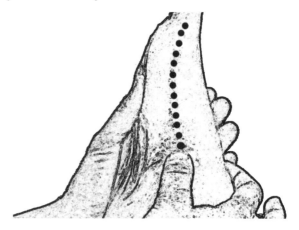

3rd Lumbar for nerve supply to the bladder.

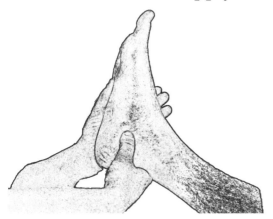 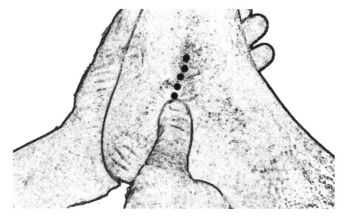

Kidney Stones- are crystals that stick together when certain chemicals form in the urine. The crystals may grow into stones. Usually the small stones can pass through the urinary system, but the larger stones block the flow of urine. Most stones contain calcium oxalate.

Direct Reflex- Kidneys

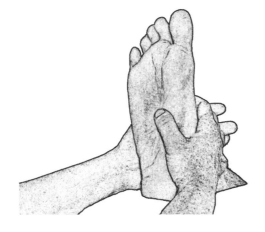 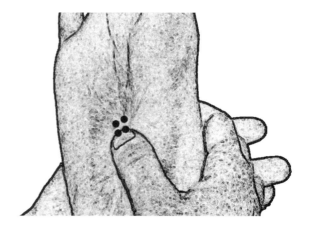

Helper Reflexes- Adrenal to strengthen muscle tone.

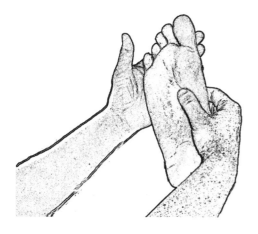 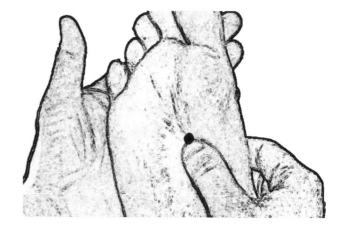

Bladder to relax the muscle to pass stones.

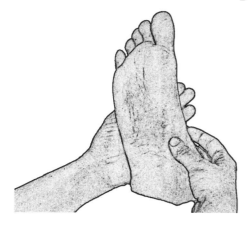 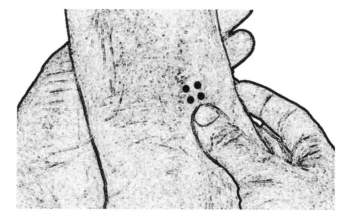

Ureter Tube to relax the muscular wall.

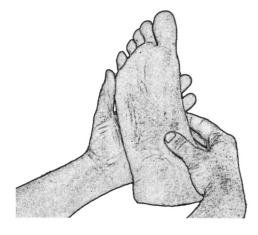 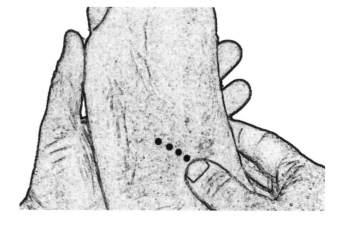

Parathyroid to control the calcium.

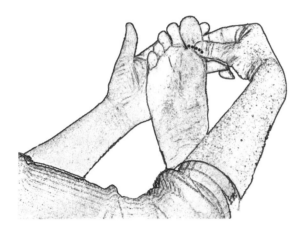 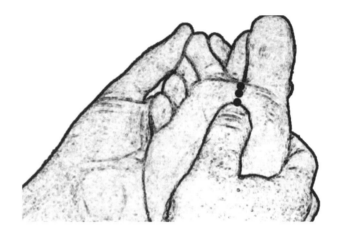

Solar Plexus to relax the body so stones can pass.

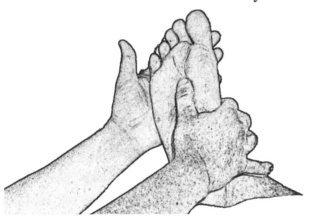 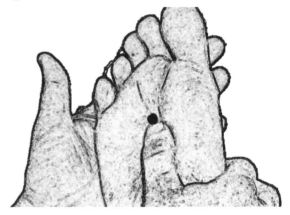

10th and 11th Thoracic better nerve supply to kidneys and ureters.

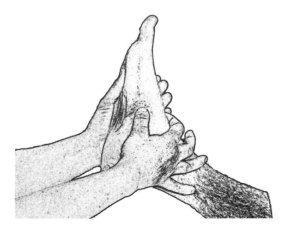 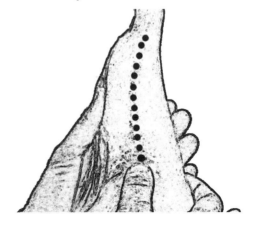

3rd Lumbar for nerve supply to the bladder.

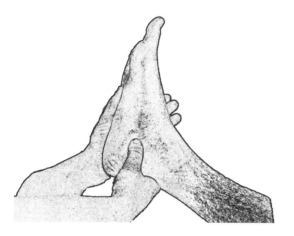 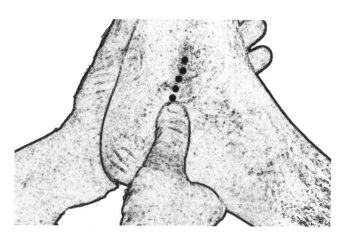

Nephritis- is inflammation of the kidneys caused by an infection.

Direct Reflex- Kidneys

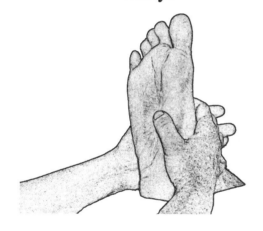 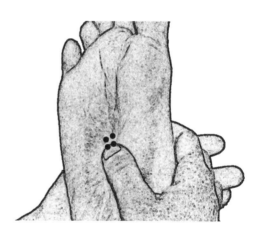

Helper Reflexes- Adrenal for inflammation.

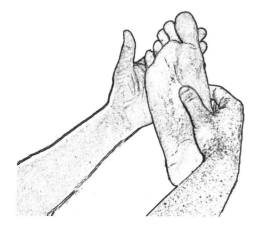 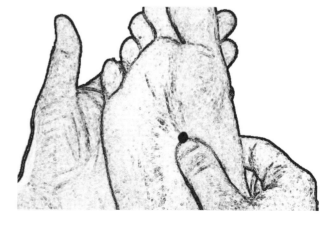

Lymphatic to help fight infection.

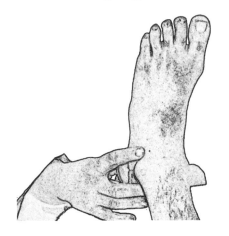 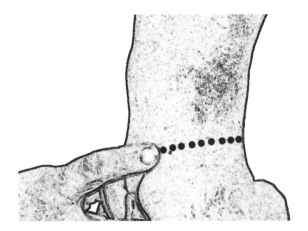

10th and 11th Thoracic for nerve supply to kidney.

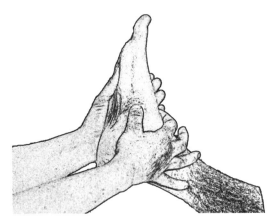 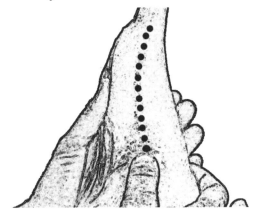

Quiz on the Urinary System

1. What function does the kidneys have in the urinary system?
   A) stores urine
   B) regulates important minerals and water
   C) manufactures vitamins and minerals

2. Where is the kidney reflex located?
   A) waistline in Zones 2 and 3 on both feet
   B) waistline in Zones 2 and 3 on the right foot
   C) diaphragm line on Zones 2 and 3 on both feet

3. What function does the bladder have in the urinary system?
   A) stores urine
   B) purifies blood
   C) retention of minerals and water

4. Where is the bladder reflex located?
   A) waistline in Zones 2 and 3
   B) medial side in Zone 1 above the heel line
   C) lateral side in Zone 5 above the heel line

5. What function does the ureter tube have in the urinary system?
   A) store urine
   B) purifies blood
   C) carry urine from kidney to bladder

6. Where is the ureter tube reflex located?
   A) in Zone 5 on the heel line
   B) in Zones 2 and 3 from the bladder to the kidney
   C) in Zone 1 at the heel line

* Answer key on page 325

Chapter 11

Respiratory System

The Respiratory System

The **Respiratory System**- consists of Lungs, Bronchial, Bronchi, Mouth, Nose, Sinuses, Trachea, Larynx, Pharynx, and Diaphragm. The function of the Respiratory system is to supply the blood with oxygen in order for the blood to deliver oxygen to every organ, gland, and other parts of the body. We inhale oxygen and exhale carbon dioxide. The gas exchange means getting oxygen to the blood.

The **Lungs**- are perhaps the most important organ of the body. The lungs are protected by the rib cage and inter-coastal muscles. The purpose of the lungs is to make the gas exchange with the outside world. The right lung is slightly larger than the left. The right lung has three lobes and the left lung two lobes. They house the bronchi and alveoli.

The reflex areas are on both feet on the plantar (bottom) side between the 2nd and 3rd, and 3rd and 4th metatarsal on the pad of the foot. Thumb-walk up from the diaphragm line to the base of the phalanges. While working this reflex you must spread the toes while thumb-walking so you can work it effectively.

The **Nose**- is the nasal entrance for air. The tiny hairs in the nasal cavity cleans and prevents foreign particles from entering the lungs. The nasal passage will moisten, filter, and warm-up the air before it reaches the lungs.

The reflex areas are on both feet on the plantar (bottom) side of the great toe about half way down. Thumb-walk from medial to lateral.

The **Para-nasal Sinuses**- are the air spaces in the bones behind your nose. The functions of the sinuses are to help regulate the temperature and humidity of air we breathe. There are four sets of sinuses that lie on each side of the nasal cavity: frontal, ethmoid, maxillary, and sphenoid sinuses.

The frontal sinuses- are located behind the bone in the forehead.

The maxillary sinuses- are located under the eyes in the cheek bones.

The ethmoid are honey-combed, and are located between the eyes.

The sphenoid sinuses are located behind the nasal cavity and behind the eyes.

The reflex areas are on both feet on the plantar (bottom) side of each small phalanges. Thumb-walk three passes down the phalanges; protect the back of toes so you have good leverage.

The **Pharynx/ Larynx-** air passes through the epiglottis, enters the pharynx (throat) and passes into the larynx (voice box). Inside the larynx is the thyroid cartilage, which surrounds the thyroid gland, and is also known as the adams apple. The larynx is very small and quickly empties into the trachea.

The reflex areas are on both feet on the plantar (bottom) side of the middle phalanges of the great toe. Thumb-walk on the medial area.

The **Trachea** (windpipe)- is the tube that connects your mouth and nose to your lungs. It is at the anterior side of the neck and is very hard, with hard rings around it. Only air passes through the trachea. Food and liquids go down the Esophagus which is located behind the trachea.

The reflex areas are on both feet on the plantar (bottom) side of the middle phalanges of the great toe. Thumb-walk on the medial area.

The **Bronchi-** the trachea divides into two cartilage ringed tubes called Bronchi. The bronchi enters the lungs and spreads into smaller tubes called Bronchial Tubes.

The reflex areas for the Bronchial are on both feet on the plantar (bottom) side between the 1st and 2nd metatarsal on the pad area. Thumb-walk up from the diaphragm line to the base of the phalanges, and spread the phalanges (toes) while walking up between the metatarsals.

The **Bronchial Tubes-** the air you breathe goes down the trachea. The bronchial tubes separate off into each lung and keep branching off into smaller tubes until the sacs at the end, called alveoli, are reached. The bronchial tubes bring the air from your trachea to your alveoli and they also help in the chore of cleaning your lungs. The bronchial tubes are covered by mucous, which holds dirt and germs that get into your lungs. The cilia has tiny hairs that clean out the debris caught in the mucous.

The reflex areas are on both feet on the plantar (bottom) side between the 1st and 2nd metatarsal on the pad area. Thumb-walk up from the diaphragm line to the base of the phalanges. Spread the phalanges while walking up between the metatarsals.

The **Alveoli-** when air enters your lungs, it goes through small tubes until it reaches tiny sacs called alveoli. The sacs looks like grapes at the end of the bronchial tubes.

The **Diaphragm** is the main muscle to draw air into the lungs. It is a muscular sheet attached to your lower ribs. It divides the chest cavity from the abdomen. It helps to pump the carbon dioxide out of the lungs and to pull oxygen into the lungs. When the diaphragm relaxes, carbon dioxide is pumped out of lungs.

The reflex areas are on both feet on the plantar (bottom) side right along the diaphragm line (under pad) from Zones 1-5. Thumb-walk medial (inside) to lateral (outside).

Diagram of the Respiratory System

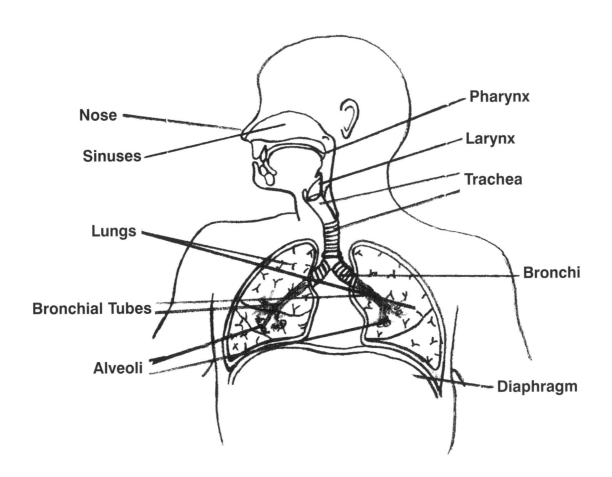

Locate the Reflex areas of the Respiratory System

*Use colored pencils to draw in reflex areas

A) Bronchial

B) Chest

C) Diaphragm

D) Lungs

E) Sinuses

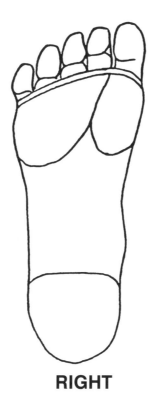

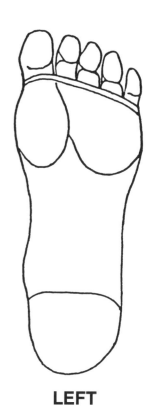

RIGHT

LEFT

TOP RIGHT

TOP LEFT

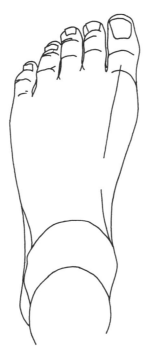

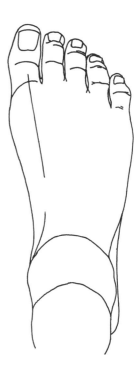

*Answer key on next page

Answer Key to the Respiratory Reflex Areas

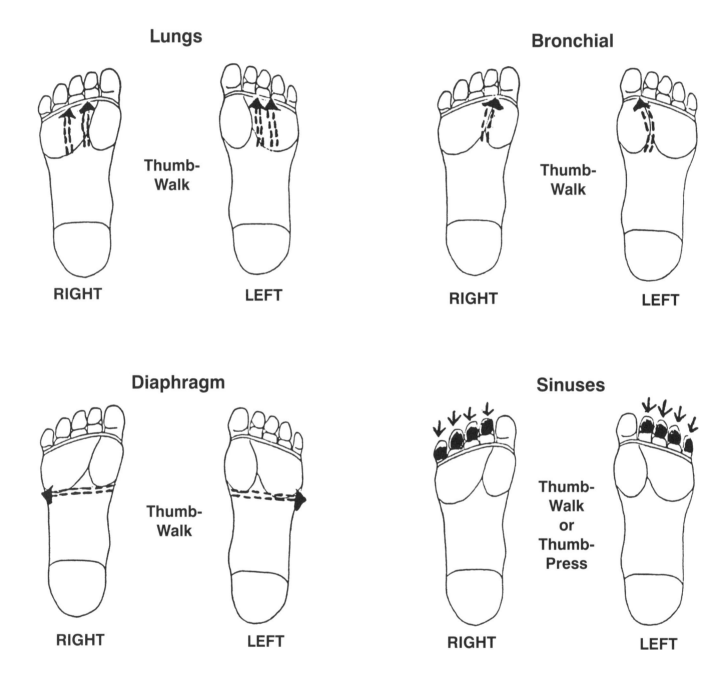

How to Work the Respiratory System Reflex Areas

The **Sinus reflex areas** are on both feet on the plantar (bottom) part of all small toes. Make at least 3-4 passes down the toes, Zones 2-5. Thumb-walk these areas.

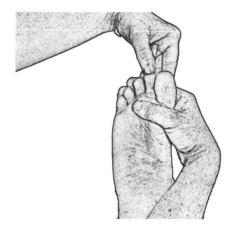
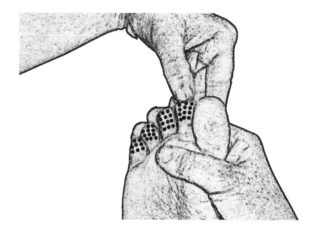

The **Bronchial Tube reflex areas** are on both feet on the plantar (bottom) part, in Zones 1 -2, spread the toes between the first and second metatarsals Thumb-walk these areas.

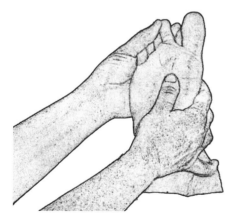
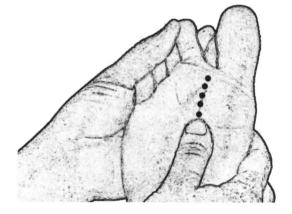

The **Lung reflex areas** are on both feet, on the plantar (bottom) part, in Zones 2 - 4 , spread the toes so you can work between the metatarsals 2 -3 and 3-4. Thumb-walk these areas.

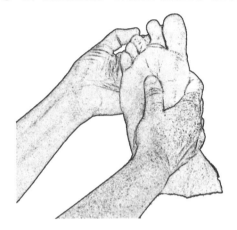 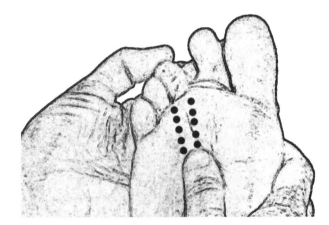

The **Diaphragm reflex areas** are on both feet on the plantar (bottom) part, in Zones 1 - 5. Thumb-walk these areas.

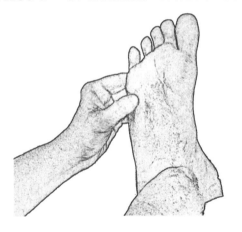 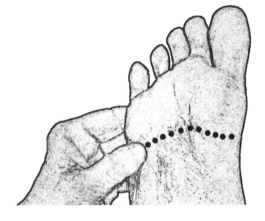

Respiratory Disorders and the Helper Reflex Areas

Allergies- are a physical disorder caused by hypersensitivity to substances that are eaten, inhaled, or come in contact with the skin.

Helper Reflexes- Adrenal suppresses inflammatory reactions.

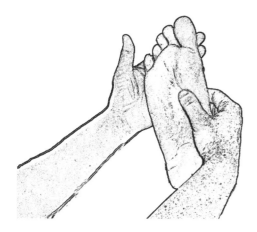
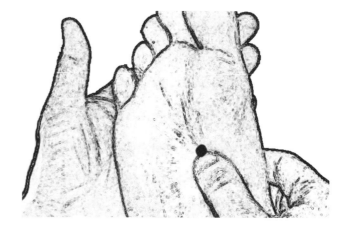

Sinuses helps to regulate the air.

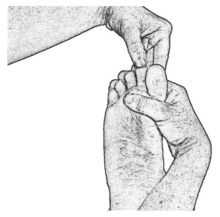
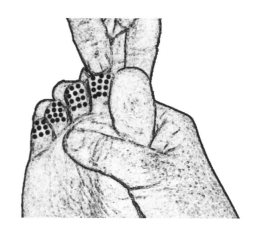

Bronchial tubes helps cleaning of lungs.

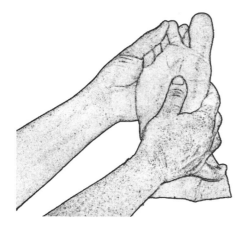
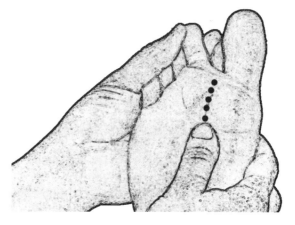

Chest/Lungs helps with getting oxygen to the blood.

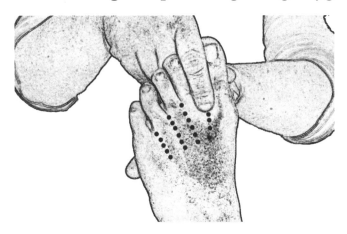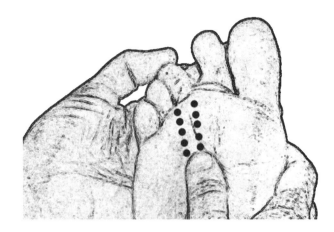

Ileocecal valve controls mucous.

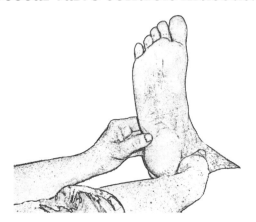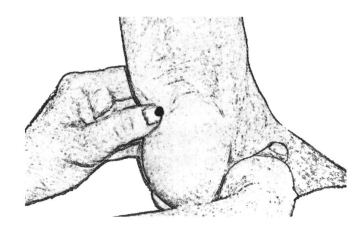

Asthma- is a chronic condition marked by periodic attacks of wheezing and difficulty in breathing. It is caused by allergies that constrict the bronchioles.

Direct Reflex- Chest/Lung helps with getting oxygen to the blood.

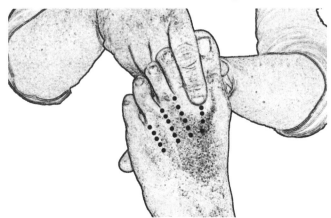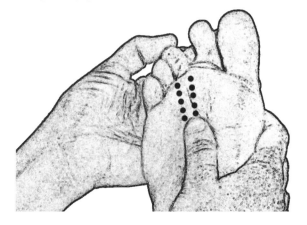

Helper Reflexes- Adrenal suppresses inflammatory reactions.

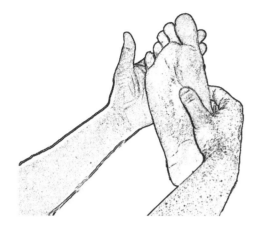
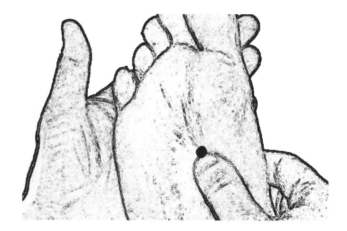

Bronchial tubes helps to clean the lungs.

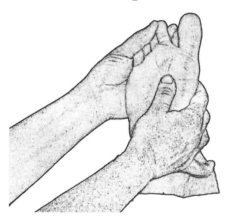
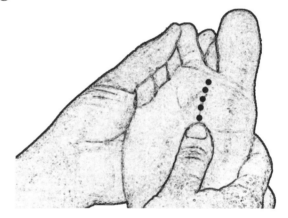

Diaphragm helps to pull oxygen into the lungs.

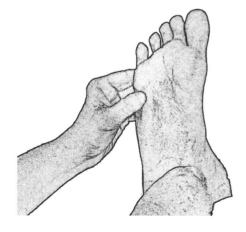
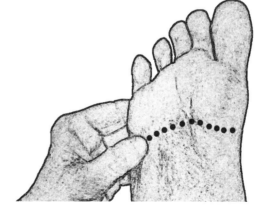

Ileocecal valve helps to control mucous.

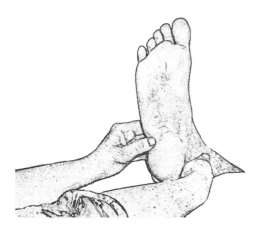
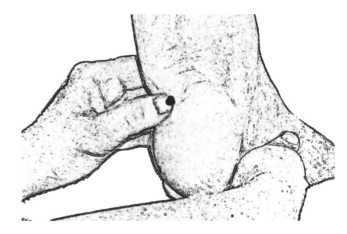

Bronchitis- is an inflammation of the bronchial tubes.

Direct Reflex- Bronchial tubes helps to clean the lungs.

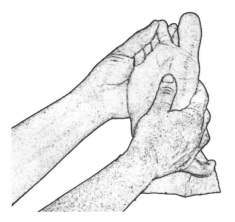
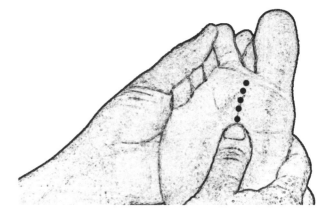

Helper Reflexes- Adrenal suppresses the inflammation.

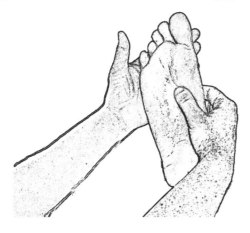
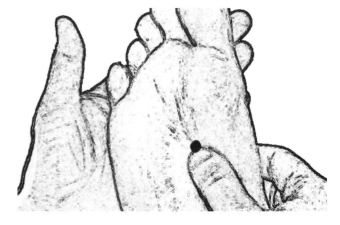

Chest/Lung helps with getting oxygen to the blood.

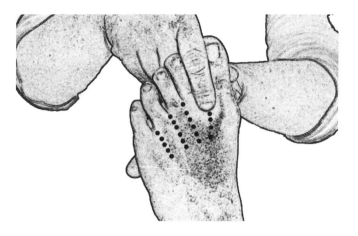 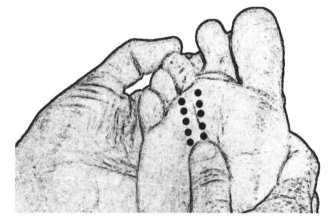

Diaphragm helps to pull oxygen into the lungs.

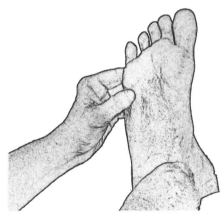 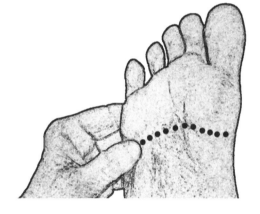

Ileocecal valve helps to control mucous.

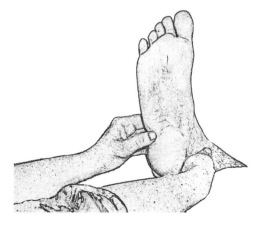 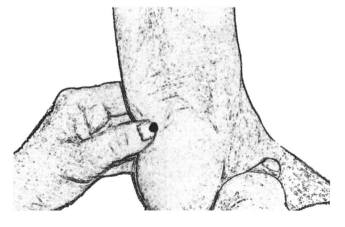

Emphysema- is a destruction of the alveolar walls.

Direct Reflex- Chest/Lungs helps to get oxygen to the lungs.

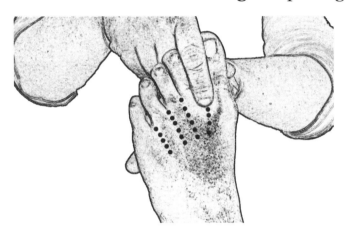 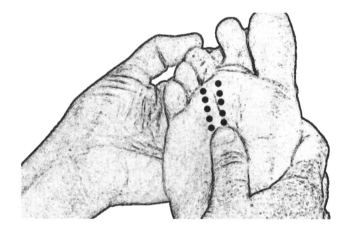

Helper Reflexes- Adrenal suppresses inflammatory reactions.

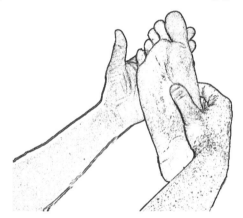 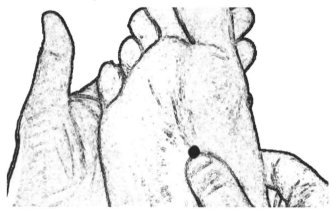

Diaphragm helps to pull oxygen into the lungs.

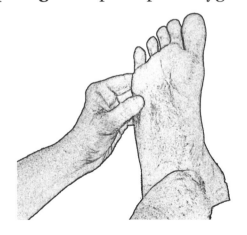 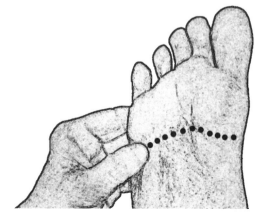

Ileocecal valve controls mucous.

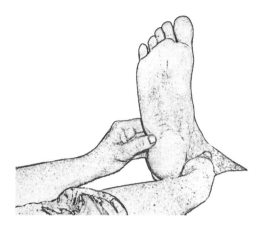
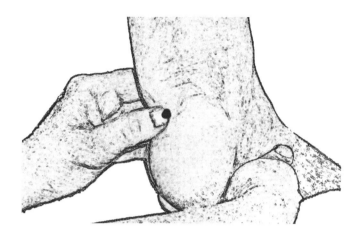

Lymphatic system helps to defend the body against diseases.

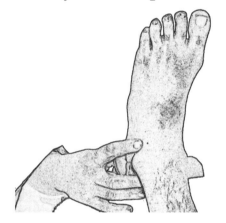
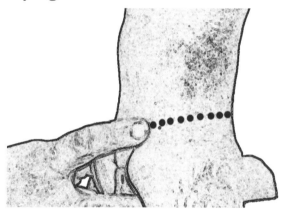

Pneumonia- is a inflammation of the lungs caused by bacteria, viruses, or chemical toxins. This infection causes the air sacs to fill with pus and other liquids.

Direct Reflex- Chest/Lung helps to get oxygen to the blood.

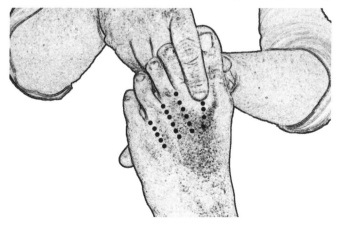
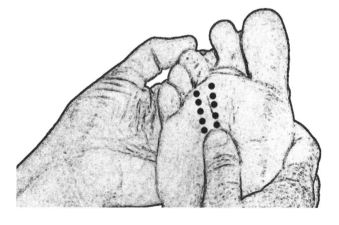

Helper Reflexes- Adrenal suppresses inflammatory reactions.

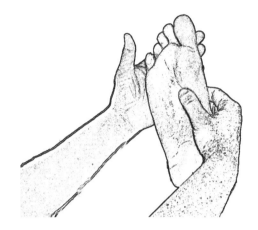
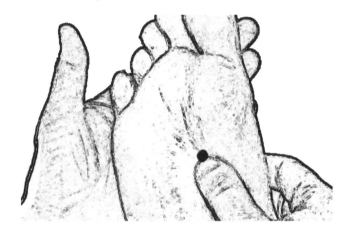

Diaphragm helps to pull oxygen into the lungs.

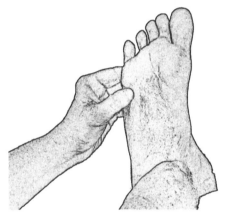
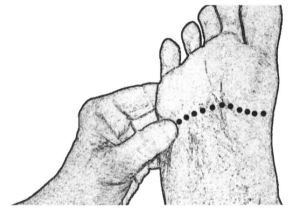

Ileocecal valve controls mucous.

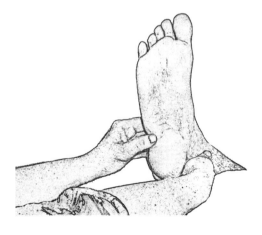
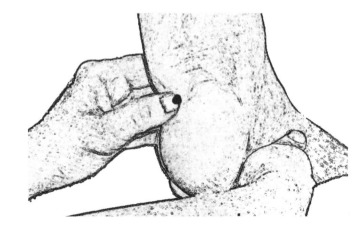

Lymphatic system defend the body against diseases.

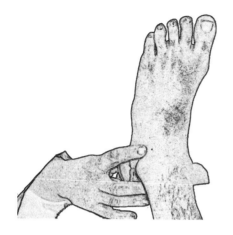 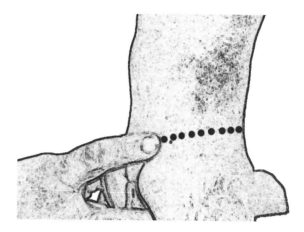

Sinusitis- is an inflammation of the mucous membranes of the sinuses.

Direct Reflex- Sinuses regulate the air we breathe.

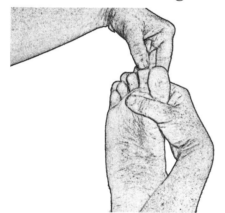  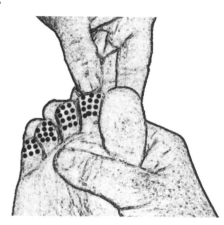

Helper Reflexes- Adrenal suppresses inflammatory reactions.

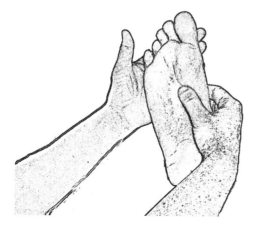 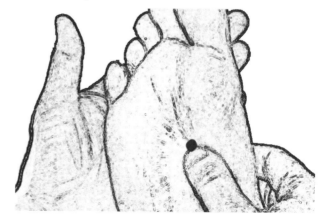

Ileocecal valve controls mucous.

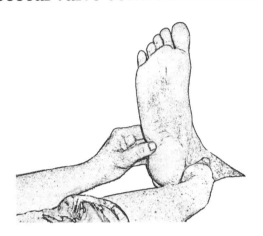
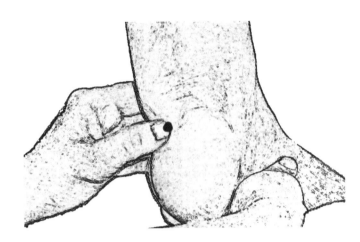

Shortness of breath- many reasons for shortness of breath. All of the above could be the culprit.

Direct Reflex- Chest/lung helps to get oxygen into the blood.

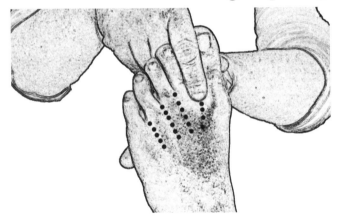
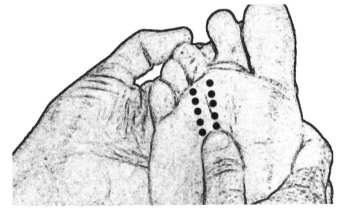

Helper Reflexes- Adrenal helps suppress inflammatory reactions.

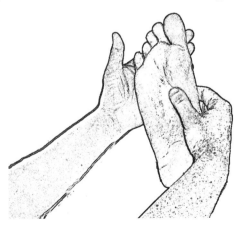
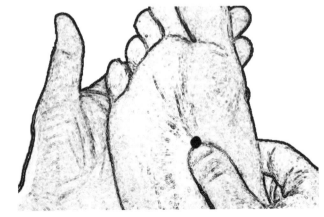

Diaphragm helps to pull oxygen into the lungs.

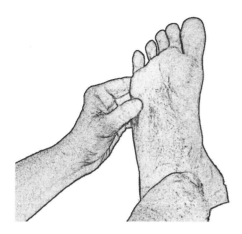 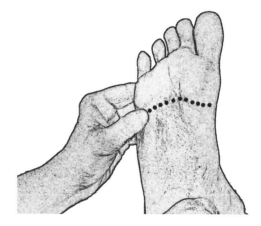

Ileocecal valve controls mucous.

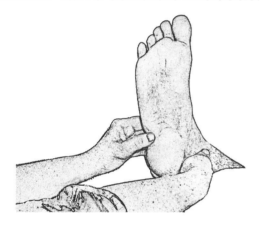 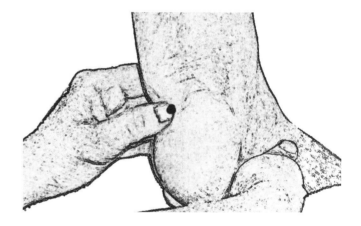

Sinuses regulates the air we breathe.

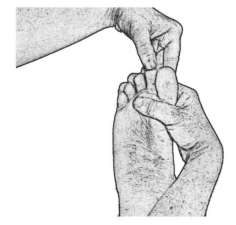 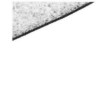 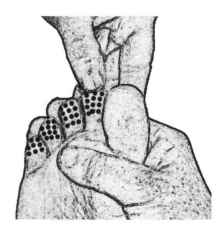

Quiz on the Respiratory System

1. What are the functions of the lungs?
   A) to make gas exchange with the outside world
   B) for the entrance of air
   C) to regulate temperature

2. Where are the lung reflex areas?
   A) all small toes   B) plantar side between first and second metatarsal
   C) plantar side between second and third, third and fourth metatarsals

3. What are the functions of the nose?
   A) entrance for air   B) to make gas exchange
   C) regulate temperature

4. Where are the nose reflex areas?
   A) all small toes   B) both great toes halfway down
   C) on the diaphragm line

5. What are the functions of the sinuses?
   A) regulate the temperature   B) entrance for air
   C) to make gas exchange

6. Where are the sinus reflex areas?
   A) both great toes halfway down   B) all small toes
   C) between the first and second metatarsal

7. What are the functions of the diaphragm?
   A) clean the lungs   B) to make gas exchange
   C) to pump carbon dioxide out of the lungs and pull in the oxygen

8. Where are the diaphragm reflex areas?
   A) between first and second metatarsal   B) on the diaphragm line
   C) all small toes

* Answer key on page 325

Chapter 12

Lymphatic System

Lymphatic System

The **Lymphatic system-** is used to help defend the body against invasion of diseases (such as viruses, bacteria, and fungi) by producing lymphocytes or white blood cells. It is a network of vessels that help in the circulation of body fluids. These vessels take excess fluid away from spaces around the cells and return it to the bloodstream.

The **Lymph nodes-** are small bean-shaped nodules and are found through out the body. The major nodes are found in the neck, groin, and armpits, and are scattered all along the lymph vessels. They have two main function; to produce white blood cells called lymphocytes that recognize bacteria and viruses, and to remove large proteins from the tissue and return them to circulation for elimination. Lymph nodes act as barriers to infection by filtering toxins and germs.

The reflex areas are found on the dorsal (top) part of both feet from medial talus to lateral talus (ankle) in Zones 1-5 and between the 1st and 2nd metatarsals on the dorsal (top) part on both feet. Finger-walk these areas.

The **Thymus** is found in front of the heart and behind the upper part of the sternum. This gland makes T-cells and lymphocytes. The thymus is huge until the person hits puberty. Then it starts to decrease in size, so that by the time a person is 50 years old the thymus is small or might be entirely gone.

The reflex areas are found on the medial (inside) part of both feet in Zone 1 between the baseline of the toes and diaphragm line. Thumb-walk this area.

The **Tonsils** are found in the back of your throat on each side. They are the first defense against air borne bacteria. Tonsils trap bacteria and viruses entering through the throat and produce antibodies to help fight infections.

The reflex areas are found on the plantar (bottom) part of the great toe on both feet about three-quarters of the way down from the tip of the toe. Thumb-walk across.

Spleen is found in the upper left part of the abdomen. It is a large lymph node. It stores iron and controls the production of red blood cells and antibodies. There are two components of the spleen, the red pulp and white pulp. The red pulp facilitates removal of old or damaged red blood cells from the circulation. The white pulp consists of lymphoid tissue and is responsible for the immunological function. It contains T-cells, B-cells, and accessory cells. The purpose of the white pulp is to mount an immunological response to antigens within the blood.

The reflex area is found on the left plantar (bottom) under the diaphragm line in Zones 4 and 5. Thumb-walk this area.

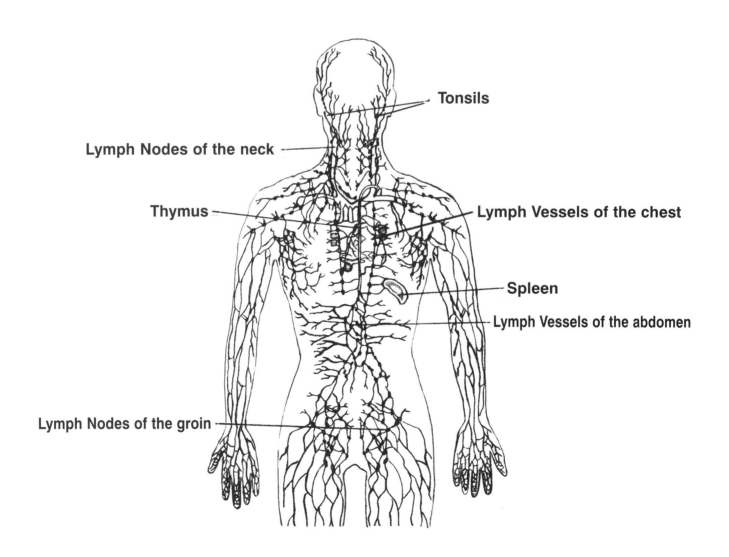

Locate the Reflex areas of the Lymphatic System

*Use colored pencils to draw in reflex areas

    A) Lymphatic System

    B) Lymph Nodes

    C) Spleen

    D) Thymus

    E) Tonsil

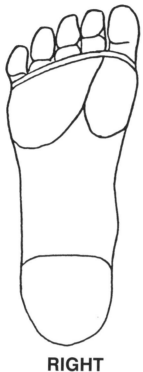
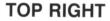

RIGHT

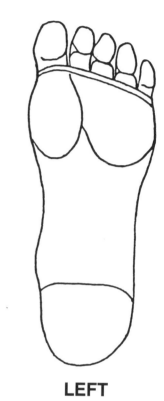

LEFT

TOP RIGHT

TOP LEFT

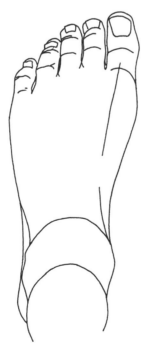
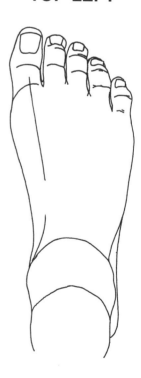

*Answer key on next page

Answer Key to the Lymphatic Reflex Areas

Tonsils

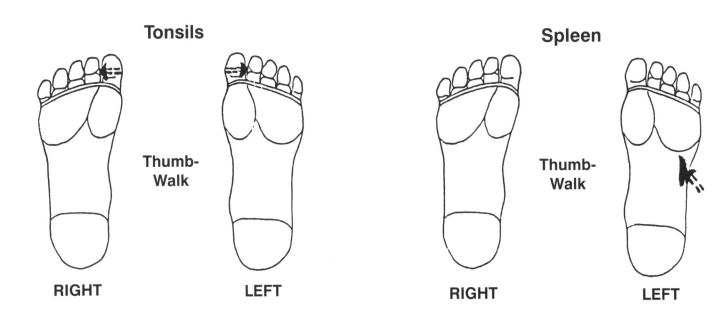

Thumb-Walk

RIGHT   LEFT

Spleen

Thumb-Walk

RIGHT   LEFT

Lymph Nodes

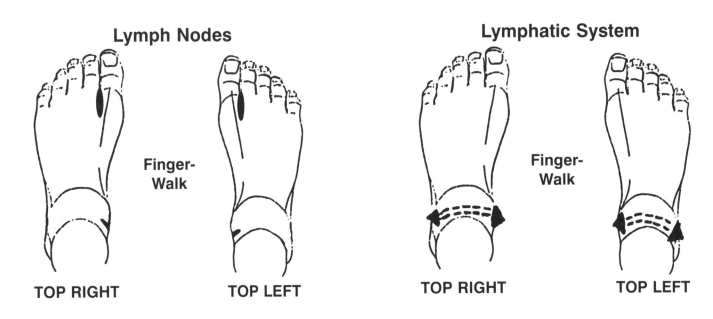

Finger-Walk

TOP RIGHT   TOP LEFT

Lymphatic System

Finger-Walk

TOP RIGHT   TOP LEFT

How to Work the
Lymphatic System Reflex Areas

The **Spleen reflex area** is on the left foot, on the plantar (bottom) part, in Zone 4-5 under the diaphragm. Thumb-walk this area.

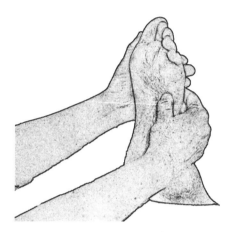 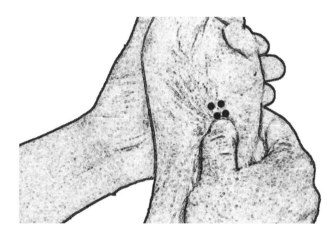

The **Tonsil reflex areas** are on both great toes, on the plantar (bottom) part, three-quarters down. Thumb-walk across these areas.

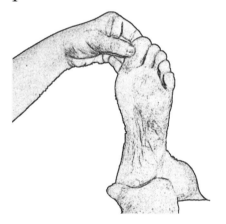 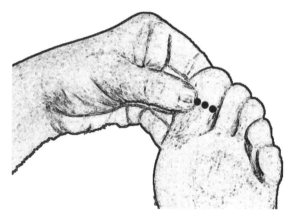

The **Lymph Nodes** under the arm reflex areas are on both feet, on the dorsal (top) part, between metatarsal 1-2. Push your fist into the ball of the foot to spread the metatarsals. Finger- walk down these areas.

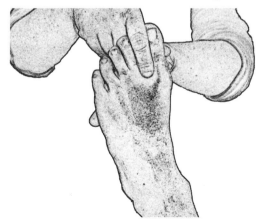 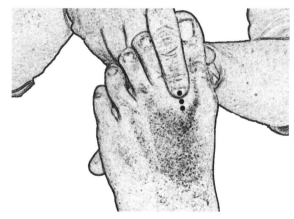

The **Lymph Nodes** in the Groin reflex areas are on both feet, on the dorsal (top) part, in Zone 1, starting at the talus (ankle) for an inch. Finger-walk these areas.

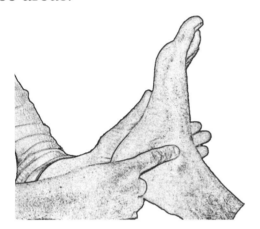 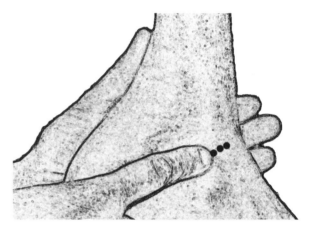

The **Lymphatic System reflex areas** are on both feet, on the dorsal (top) part, in Zones 1-5, starting from medial (inside) at the talus (ankle) to the lateral (outside) talus (ankle). Finger-walk these areas.

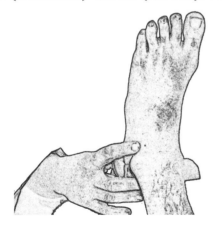 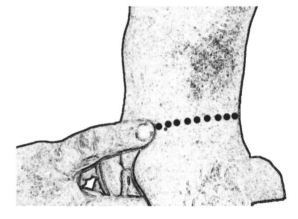

Lymphatic Disorders and the Helper Reflex Areas

Anemia- occurs when the blood does not have enough hemoglobin. Hemoglobin is a protein in the red blood cells that carries oxygen from the lungs to the rest of the body. Anemia can be an iron deficiency.

Direct Reflex- Spleen it helps to control the production of red blood cells.

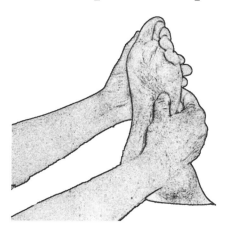 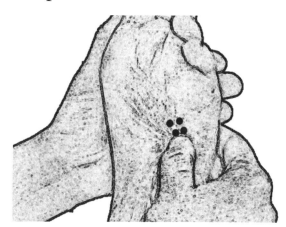

Helper Reflexes- Liver it detoxifies the blood.

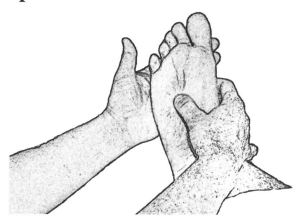 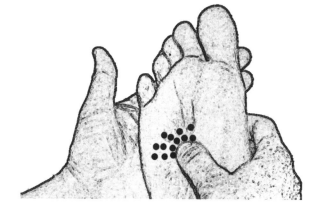

The Immune System- is a complex system of organs, special cells, and a circulatory system separate from blood vessels, which work together to clear infection from the body.

Direct Reflex- Thymus to make T-cells.

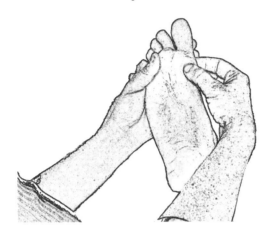 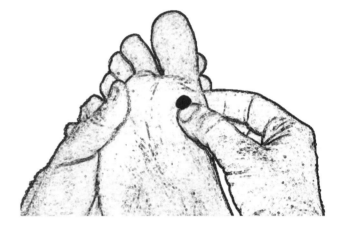

Helper Reflexes- Lymphatic system it helps the invasion of diseases.

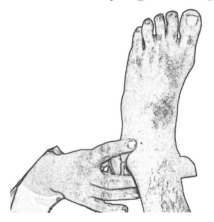 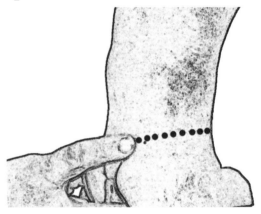

Lymphoedema- is a swelling caused by an interruption of the normal drainage of lymph back into the blood.

Direct Reflex- Lymphatic System it takes the excess fluid away from spaces around the cells.

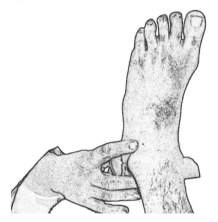
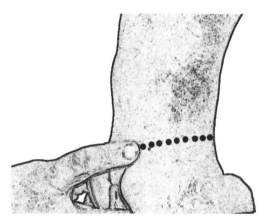

Lymphoma- cancer cells of the lymphatic system. The lymph vessels, lymph nodes, tonsils, and spleen are involved in fighting the infection.

Direct Reflex- Lymphatic System defends the body against invasion of diseases.

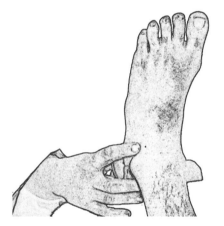
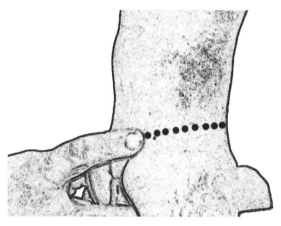

Helper Reflexes- Tonsil they are the first defense against diseases.

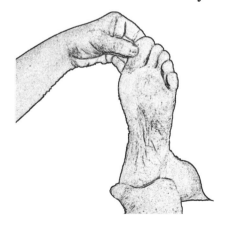
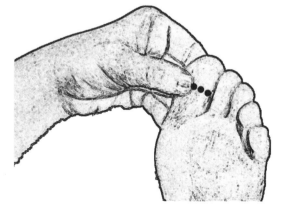

Spleen controls production of antibodies.

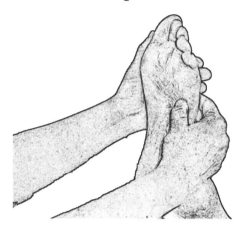 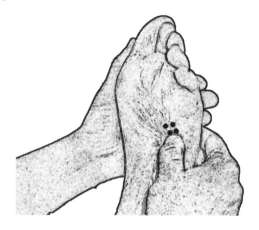

Raynauds Disease- is a disorder that constricts the blood vessels in the fingers, toes, ears, and nose.

Direct Reflex- Lymphatic system it has a network of vessels that helps with the circulation of body fluids. *Also work the affected area.

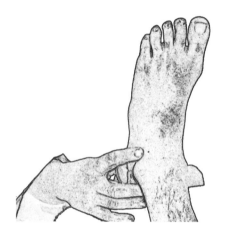 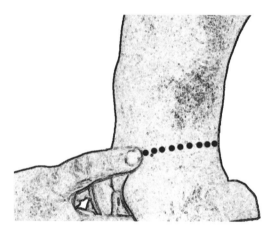

Tonsillitis- swollen tonsils caused by an infection.

Direct Reflex- Tonsils first defense in airborne diseases.

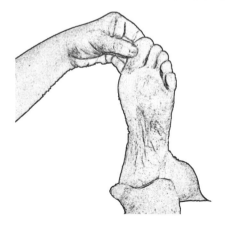 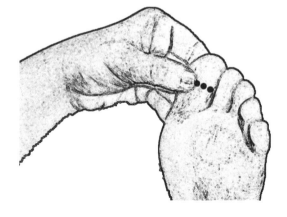

Helper Reflexes- Adrenal for the inflammation.

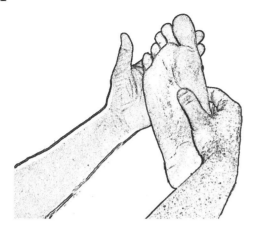 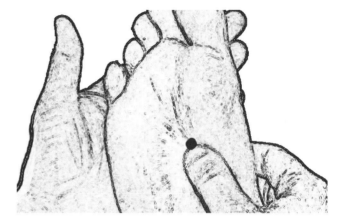

Lymphatic System defends the body from airborne diseases.

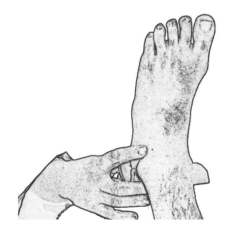 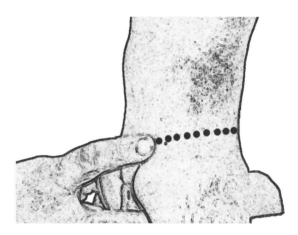

All Neck Reflexes for better blood and nerve supply.

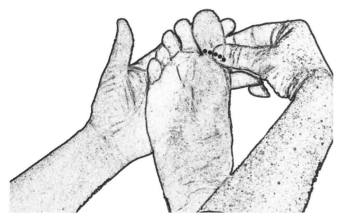 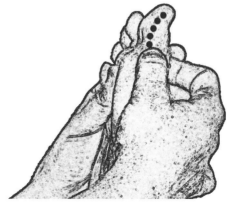

Quiz on the Lymphatic System

1. What is the function of the thymus?
   A) makes T-cells and lymphocytes
   B) remove large proteins from the tissues
   C) defends airborne diseases

2. Where are the thymus reflex areas located?
   A) top of the feet from ankle to ankle
   B) medial side in Zone 1 on both feet between baseline of
      the toes and diaphragm line
   C) on them left foot plantar side under the diaphragm line in Zones 4 and 5

3. What is the function of the lymph nodes?
   A) makes T-cells and lymphocytes
   B) to remove large proteins from the tissue
   C) stores iron and controls the production of red blood cells

4. Where are the lymph node reflex areas?
   A) great toe three- quarters of the way down
   B) top of the feet from ankle to ankle
   C) left plantar under diaphragm line in Zones 4 and 5

5. What is the function of the spleen?
   A) to make T-cells and lymphocytes
   B) stores iron and controls the production of
      red blood cells and antibodies
   C) to produce white blood cells

6. Where is the spleen reflex area?
   A) left plantar under the diaphragm line in Zones 4 and 5
   B) great toe three-quarters of the way down
   C) top of feet from ankle to ankle

* Answer key on page 325

Chapter 13

Hip,
Knee,
Shoulder,
Elbow,
and Wrist

Hip, Knee, Leg, Shoulder, Elbow, and Wrist

The **Hip-** consists of two coxal bones. The hip is a place of muscle attachment for the back, abdomen, hamstrings, quadriceps, abductors, adductors, and gluteal muscles. Most of the muscles are shorter to allow for rotation and stabilization of the joint.

The reflex area of the hip is found on the lateral (outside) of the foot on both feet between the cuboid and calcaneous. Thumb or finger-walk in the triangle area on both feet. Also use the thumb-walking around lateral (outside) ankle bone if the hip pain is chronic.

The **Knee-** consists of ligaments, tendons, and bones. The three main bones are the Femur (thigh bone), the longest and strongest bone in the body, the tibia (lower leg bone), the second largest bone in the body, (the weight bearing bone of the leg), and the patella (knee cap), which protects the knee joint. There are two ligaments the medial collateral and lateral collateral on each side of the knee.

The reflex area is found on the lateral (outside) of the foot between the cuboid and calcaneous in the triangle area on both feet. Thumb or finger-walk the area.

The **Shoulder-** consist of two bones-the clavicle (collar bone) and the scapula (shoulder blade). The shoulder has several layers, the deepest are the bones and the joints, then the ligaments, tendons, and muscles.

The reflex area is found on the plantar side in the 5th Zone on the diaphragm line on both feet. Thumb-walk this area.

The **Elbow-**is formed by three bones, the humerous, radius, and ulna. The main function is to position and stabilize the hand. These three bones come together to move in flexion, extension, and rotation.

The reflex area is found between the 4th and 5th metatarsal, between the diaphragm line and toe line halfway up on both feet. Thumb-walk this area.

The **Wrist**- consists of eight carpal bones that form the carpal tunnel, which is located between the forearm and the hand. The carpal tunnel allows for the many motions of the wrist.

The reflex area is found between the 4th and 5th metatarsal between the diaphragm line and the toe line three-quarters up near the toe line on both feet. Thumb-walk this area.

Diagram of Shoulder, Elbow, and Wrist

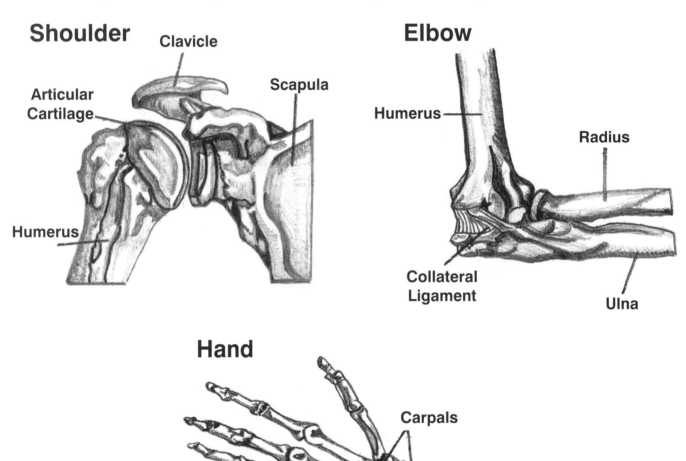

Diagram of Hip and Knee

Hip

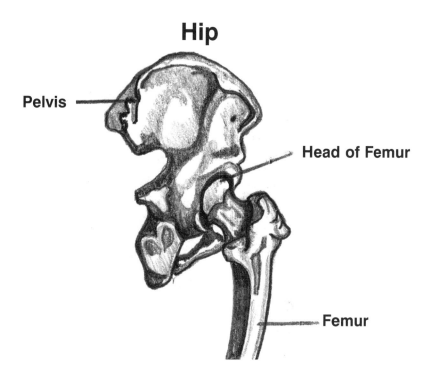

Pelvis

Head of Femur

Femur

Knee

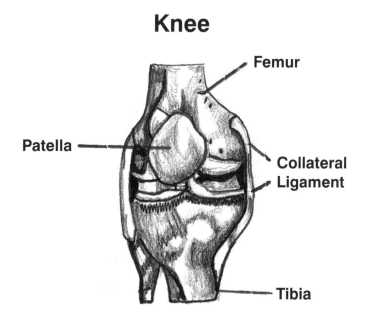

Femur

Patella

Collateral Ligament

Tibia

Locate the Reflex areas of the Hip, Knee, Leg, Shoulder, and Wrist

*Use colored pencils to draw in reflex areas

    A) Hip

    B) Knee

    C) Leg

    D) Shoulder

    E) Elbow

    F) Wrist

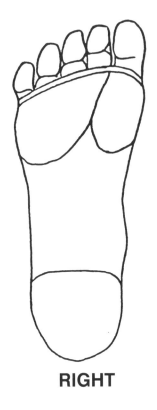

RIGHT

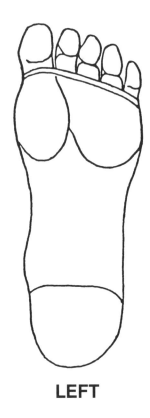

LEFT

INSIDE

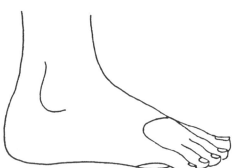

OUTSIDE

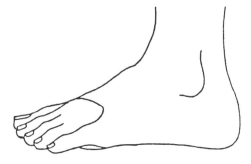

*Answer key on next page

Answer Key to the Hip, Knee, Shoulder Reflex Areas

Hip

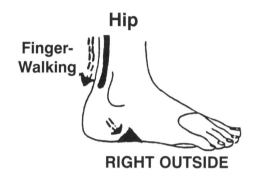

Finger-Walking

RIGHT OUTSIDE

Knee

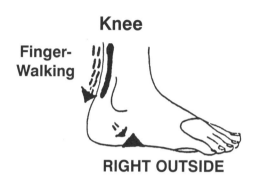

Finger-Walking

RIGHT OUTSIDE

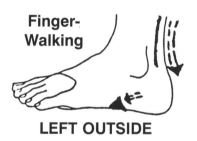

Finger-Walking

LEFT OUTSIDE

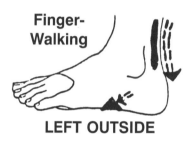

Finger-Walking

LEFT OUTSIDE

Leg

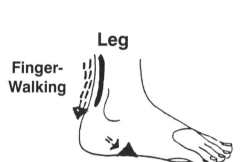

Finger-Walking

RIGHT OUTSIDE

Knee

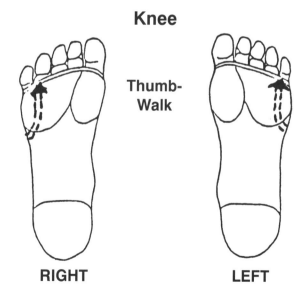

Thumb-Walk

RIGHT   **LEFT**

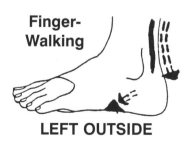

Finger-Walking

LEFT OUTSIDE

How to Work the Hip, Knee, Shoulder Reflex Areas

The **Hip/Knee/Leg reflex areas** are on both feet, on the lateral (outside) part, in Zone 5, between the calcaneus (heel) and the third cuboid bone. Finger-walk these areas.

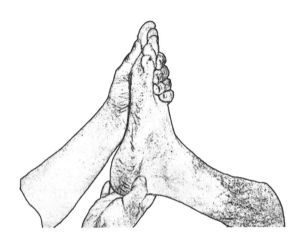 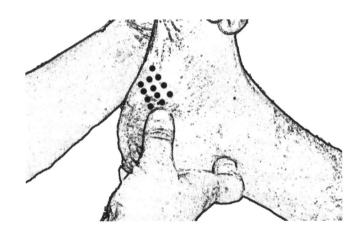

The **Chronic Hip/Knee/Leg reflex areas** are on the lateral (outside) of each leg. Thumb-walk down to around the talus (ankle).

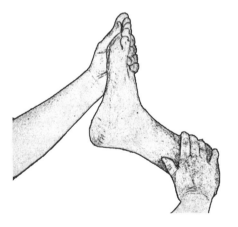 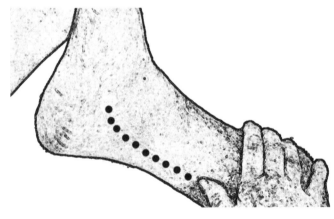

The **Shoulder reflex areas** are on both feet, on the plantar (bottom) part, in Zone 5, on the diaphragm line, and between metatarsal 4 - 5. Thumb-walk these areas.

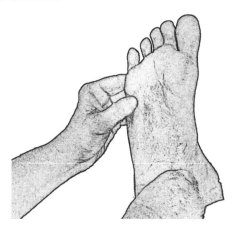 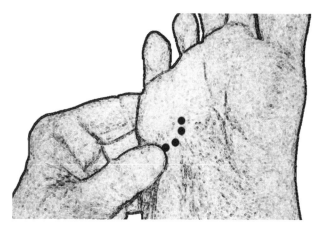

The **Elbow reflex areas** are on both feet, on the plantar (bottom) part, between Zones 4 - 5, spread the toes so you can get between metatarsal 4 - 5. Thumb-walk these areas.

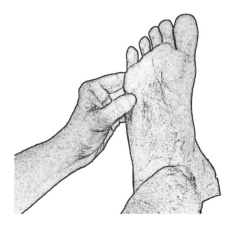 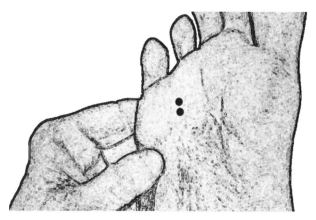

The **Wrist reflex areas** are on both feet, on the plantar (bottom) part, in Zones 4 - 5. Spread the toes so you can get between the metatarsals 4 - 5. Thumb-walk these areas.

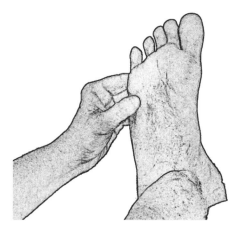 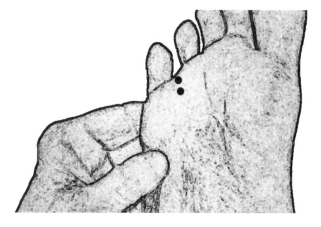

Hip, Knee, Leg, and Shoulder, Elbow, Wrist Disorders and the Helper Reflex Areas

Pain in Hip, Knee- may involve a wide variety of problems.

Direct Reflex- Hip or knee

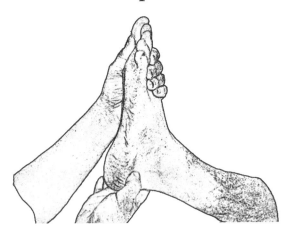
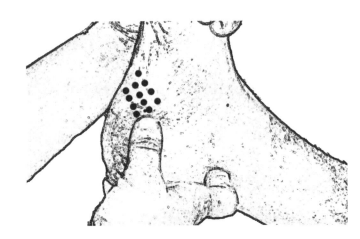

Referral Reflex- If in the hip, you would work the shoulder - if in the knee, work the elbow.

Helper Reflexes- Adrenal suppress inflammation.

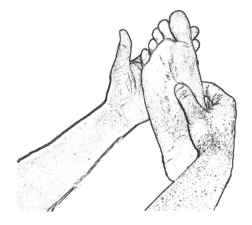
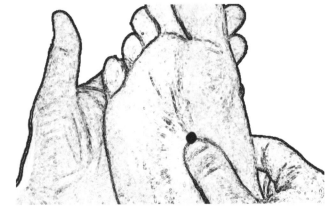

3rd Lumbar for knees for better blood and nerve supply.

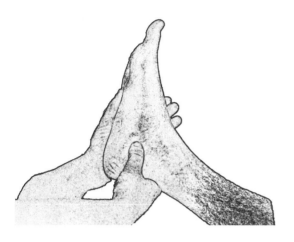 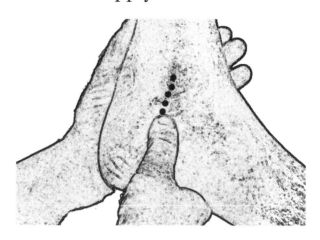

Sacral for hip for better blood and nerve supply.

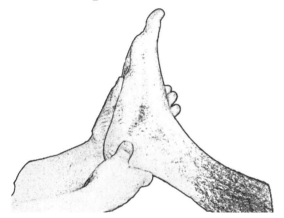 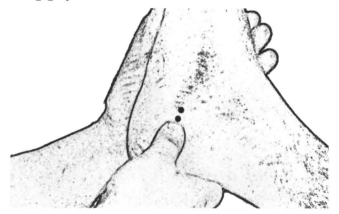

Carpal Tunnel Syndrome- the carpal tunnel is a bony canal on the palm side of the hand and the median nerve goes through it to the hand. Pinching of this nerve causes pain, numbness, inflammation, tingling of the hand, and weakness of the grip.

Direct Reflex- Wrist

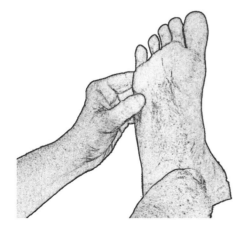 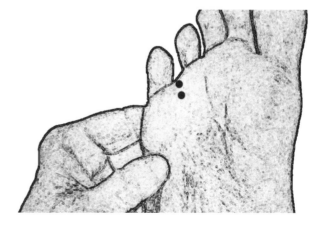

Referral Reflex- Ankle

Helper Reflexes- Adrenal suppresses inflammation.

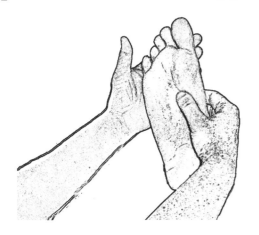
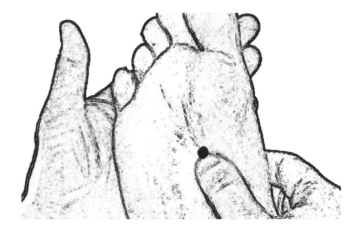

1st Thoracic helps to get better blood and nerve supply.

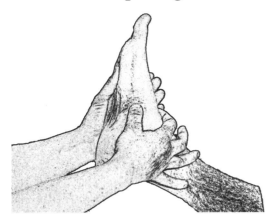
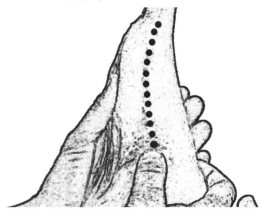

* Work directly on the hands thumb-walking up from wrist up to phalanges, work up all the zones.

Sprained Ankle or Wrist - is a stretched or torn ligament (the ligaments hold bones together), which causes pain and swelling.

Strained Ankle or Wrist - is an injury to the muscles or tendons (connects muscle to bone). It is caused by over-use.

Referral Reflex- if ankle, work the wrist; if wrist, work the ankle.

Tennis Elbow - an inflammation when the outer part of the elbow becomes painful and tender, usually it is caused by a strain (overuse of the muscle), or a direct injury.

Direct Reflex- Elbow

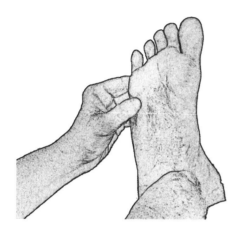 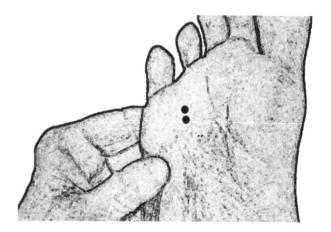

Helper Reflexes - Adrenal suppresses inflammation.

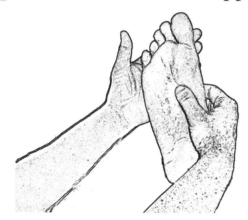 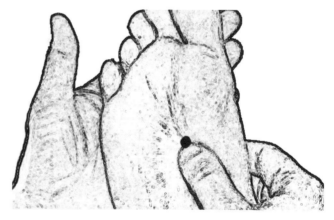

7th Cervical for better blood and nerve supply.

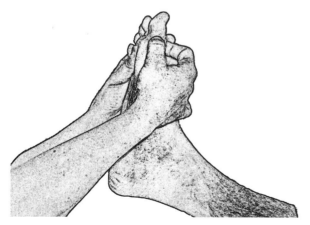 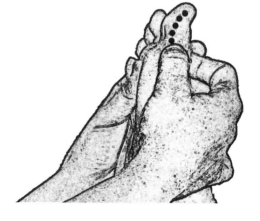

Quiz on the Hip, Knee, Shoulder, Elbow, and Wrist

1. The hip and knee reflex is located where?
   A) medial side in Zone 1 above the heel line
   B) lateral, plantar side above the heel line
   C) lateral side between the cuboid and calcaneous

2. If the hip is injured what referral area would you have to work?
   A) elbow   B) shoulder   C) wrist

3. The shoulder reflex is located where?
   A) medial side in Zone 1 at the diaphragm line
   B) lateral side in Zone 5 at the diaphragm line
   C) plantar side in Zone 3 at the diaphragm line

4. If the shoulder is injured what referral area would you work?
   A) knee   B) ankle   C) hip

5. The elbow reflex is located where?
   A) between the 4th and 5th metatarsal halfway from the diaphragm line and toe line
   B) between the 1st and 2nd metatarsal above the diaphragm line
   C) between the 2nd and 3rd metatarsal above the diaphragm line

6. If the elbow is injured what referral area would you work?
   A) knee   B) hip   C) ankle

7. The wrist reflex is located where?
   A) between the 1st and 2nd metatarsal above the diaphragm line
   B) between the 4th and 5th metatarsal above the diaphragm line three-quarters of the way near the toe line
   C) between the 3rd and 4th metatarsal above the diaphragm line

8. If the wrist is injured what referral area would you work?
   A) ankle   B) knee   C) hip

* Answer key on page 325

Chapter 14

14

Reproductive System

Reproductive System

The **Reproductive System-** are organs that produce offspring. The female reproductive organs produce female cells (the egg or ova) and include the uterus in which the development of the fetus takes place. The male reproductive system produces cells (sperm) and contains the organ that discharges the sperm into the female.

Female Reproductive

The **Uterus-** is a pear shaped organ that is located at the front of the lower abdomen, behind the bladder. It is anchored in position by six ligaments. The development of the fetus takes place here. Its walls are powerful muscles to help push out the baby during childbirth. It also contains nutrients to nourish the baby during pregnancy.

The reflex areas are found on the medial (inside) part of both feet between the talus (ankle) and calcaneus (heel). On a diagonal from the back of the heel to the ankle bone, it is located halfway between. Thumb-press this area. If the uterus has chronic problems, the reflex area are on the medial side of both legs down the tibia bone. Thumb -walk approximately six inches down.

The **Ovaries-** are located on each side of the spinal column, just above the pubic bone. The ovaries produce ova (eggs) and female hormones (estrogen and progesterone), which are responsible for female development. Each ovary holds thousands of tiny egg follicles the clusters of cells that contain immature eggs.

The reflex areas are found on the lateral (outside) part of both feet between the talus (ankle) and the calcaneus (heel). On a diagonal from the back of the heel and the ankle bone, it is located halfway. Thumb-press this area.

The **Fallopian Tubes or Uterine Tubes-** are a pair of four inch long tubes that are passageways for the egg as it travels from the ovaries to the uterus.

The reflex areas are found on the dorsal (top) part of both feet from medial (inside) talus (ankle) to lateral talus. Finger-walk this area.

The **Mammary Gland or Breast-** there is one pair of breasts and their function is to produce milk. The milk formation is stimulated by hormones. The breasts after pregnancy are made up of a system of ducts (to carry milk to the nipples) that is surrounded by glandular and fatty tissue.

The reflex areas are found on the dorsal (top) part of both feet between all the metatarsals. Finger-walk down all these areas, make a fist and put it on the ball of the foot (that spreads the metatarsals) then with your working hand finger-walk down between each metatarsal.

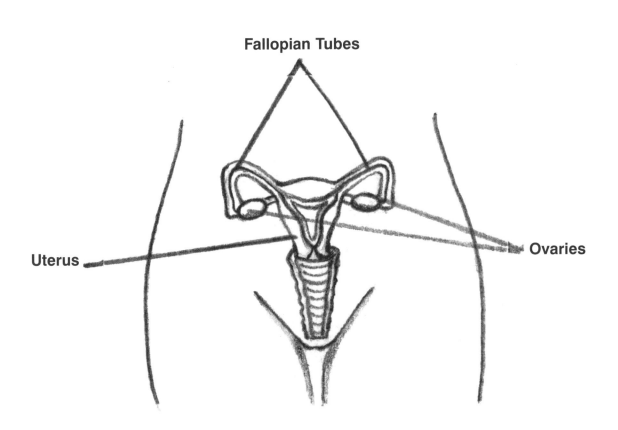

Male Reproductive

The **Prostate** is a cluster of small glands that surround the urethra. It is located in the pelvic cavity in the front of the rectum and below the bladder. It secretes the fluid part of the semen.

The reflex areas are located on the medial (inside) part of both feet between the talus (ankle) and the calcaneus (heel). On a diagonal from the back of the heel to the ankle bone, it is located halfway. Thumb-press this area. If a swollen prostate is chronic, the reflex area is on the medial side of both legs down on the side of the tibia bone. Thumb-walk down for approximately six inches.

The **Testes** are two glands in the scrotum that produce sperm and the male hormone testosterone.

The reflex areas are located on the lateral (outside) part of both feet between the talus (ankle) and the calcaneus (heel). It is located halfway on a diagonal from the back of the heel to the ankle bone. Thumb-press this area.

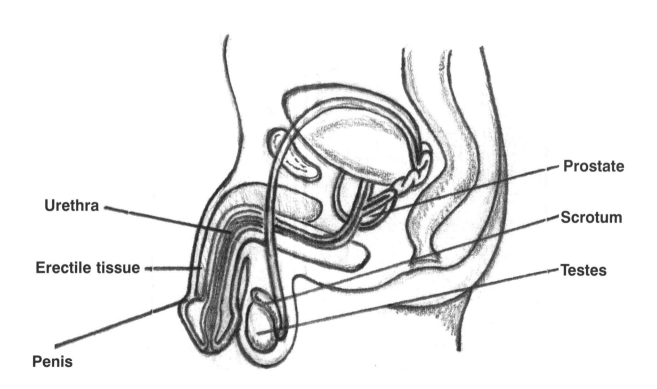

Locate the Reflex areas of the Reproductive System

Female
   A) Breast
   B) Fallopian Tube
   C) Ovary
   D) Uterus
   E) Chronic Uterus

Male
   A) Prostate
   B) Testes
   C) Chronic Prostate

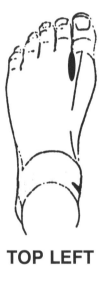 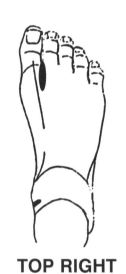

TOP LEFT   **TOP RIGHT**

INSIDE   **OUTSIDE**

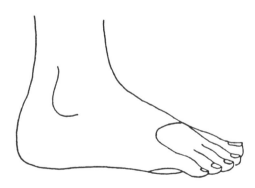 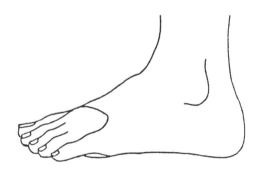

*Answer key on next page

Answer Key to the Female Reproductive Reflex Areas

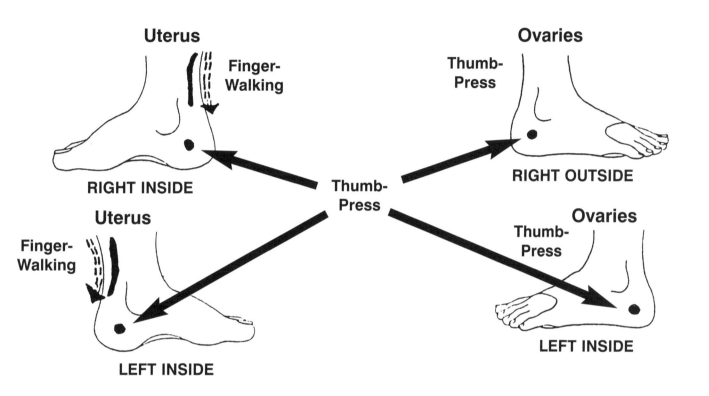

Uterus — Finger-Walking — **RIGHT INSIDE**

Uterus — Finger-Walking — **LEFT INSIDE**

Thumb-Press

Ovaries — Thumb-Press — **RIGHT OUTSIDE**

Ovaries — Thumb-Press — **LEFT INSIDE**

Fallopian Tubes

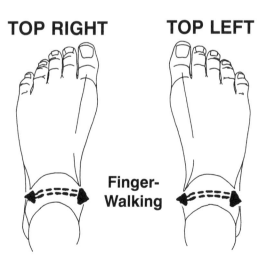

TOP RIGHT **TOP LEFT**

Finger-Walking

Breast

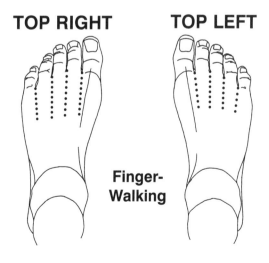

TOP RIGHT **TOP LEFT**

Finger-Walking

Answer Key to the
Male Reproductive Reflex Areas

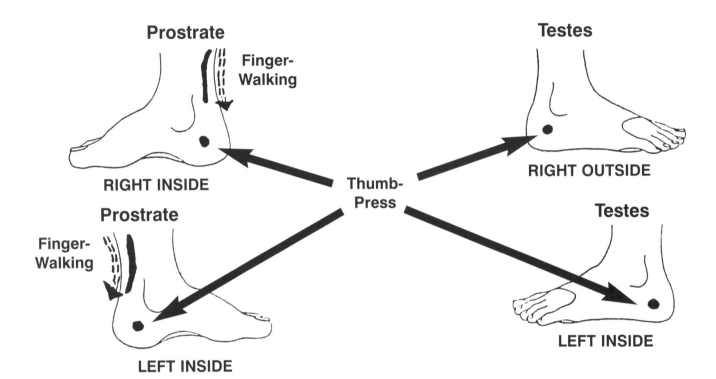

How to Work the Reproductive Reflex Areas

The **Breast reflex** areas are on both feet, on the dorsal (top) part of the foot between all the metatarsals in Zones 1-2, 2-3, 3-4, 4-5. Push your fist on the plantar (bottom) side to spread the metatarsals. Finger-walk these areas.

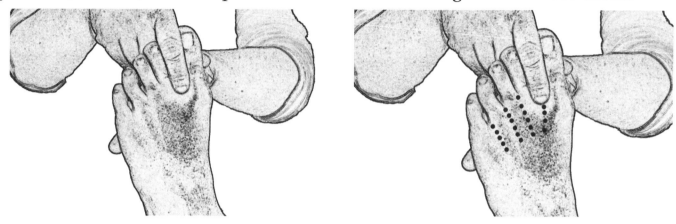

The **Fallopian Tube reflex areas** are on both feet, on the dorsal (top) part, in Zones 1-5, from talus (ankle) to talus (ankle). Finger-walk these areas.

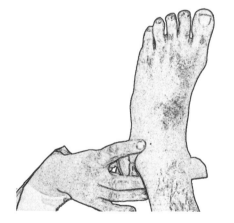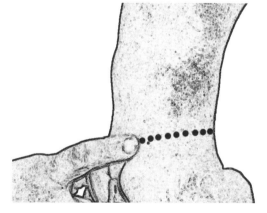

The **Ovary/Testes reflex areas** are on both feet on the lateral (outside) part, in Zone 5, between the calcaneous (heel) and the talus (ankle). Thumb-press these areas.

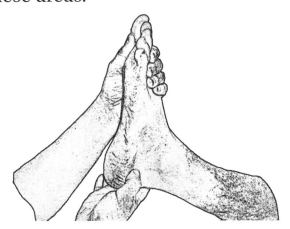 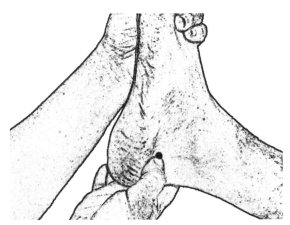

The **Uterus/ Prostate reflex areas** are on both feet, on the medial (inside) part, in Zone 1, between the calcaneous (heel) and the talus (ankle). Thumb-press these areas.

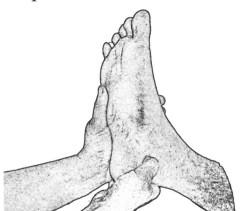 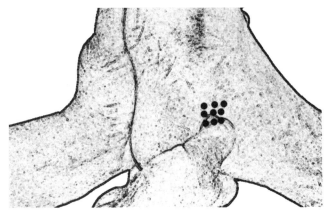

The **Chronic Uterus/Prostate reflex areas** are on both legs on the medial (inside) part, in Zone 1. Thumb-press these areas.

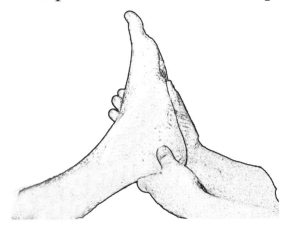 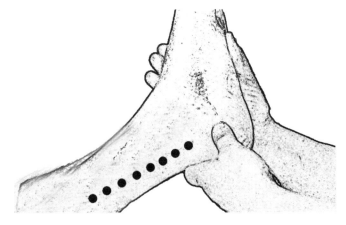

Female Reproductive Disorders and the Helper Reflex Areas

Hot Flashes- seem to be the changing of hormonal levels.

Direct Reflex- Hypothalamus helps to release hormones for emotions.

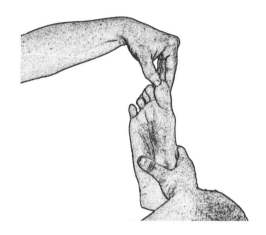 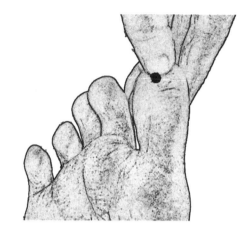

Helper Reflexes- Adrenal helps to release an adrenaline hormone for emotional stress.

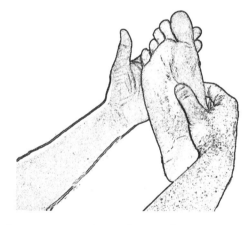 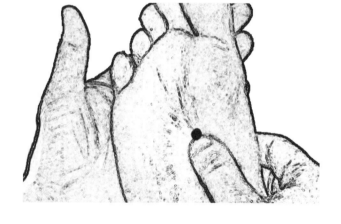

Pituitary to stimulate the ovary.

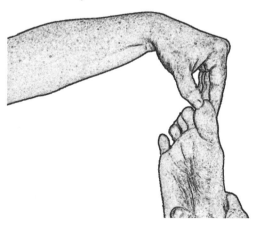 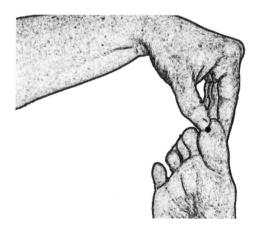

Ovary helps to release estrogen and progesterone.

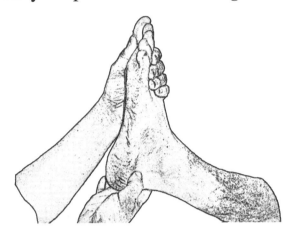
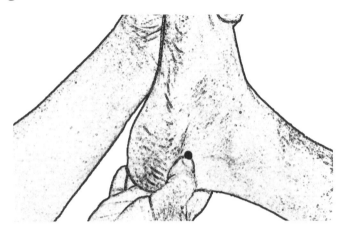

Thyroid helps to release thyroxine to regulate the body's metabolism.

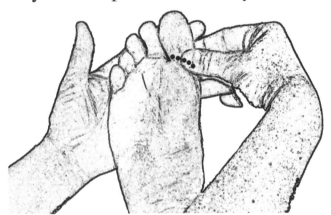
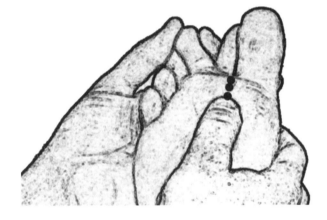

Solar plexus helps to ease stress and tension.

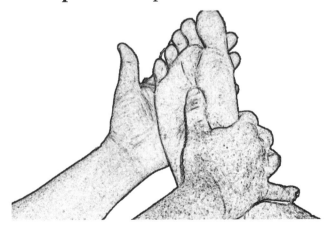
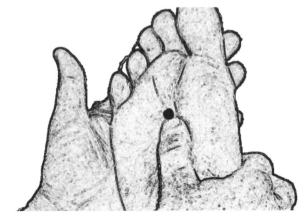

Menopause- is the end of menstrual bleeding due to a depletion of ovarian follicles (eggs).

Direct Reflex- Hypothalamus helps to release hormones for emotions.

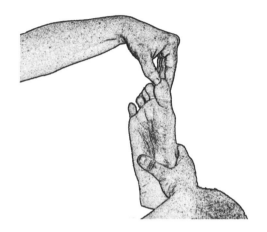 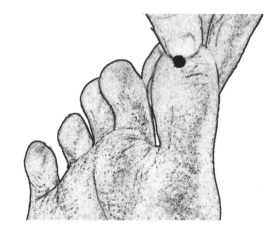

Helper Reflexes- Adrenal helps to release adrenaline for emotional stress.

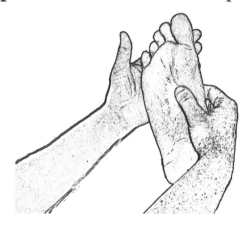 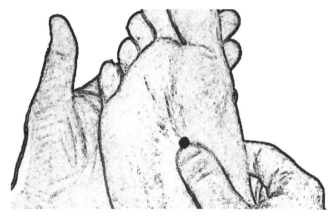

Ovaries helps to release estrogen and progesterone.

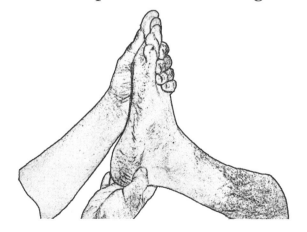 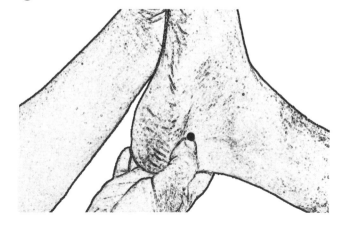

Thyroid helps to release thyroxine for the body's metabolism.

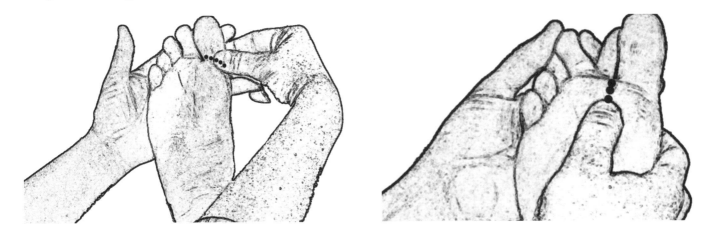

Solar Plexus helps to ease stress and tension..

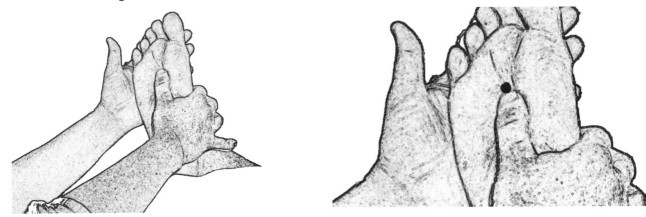

Menstrual cramping- each month the lining of the uterus gets ready for possible pregnancy. If the egg is not fertilized the lining is not needed. It breaks down and hormones are released. These trigger the muscles of the uterus to contract and squeeze the lining out. This may cause painful muscle spasms.

Direct Reflex- Uterus helps with the break down of the uterus lining and the releasing of hormones.

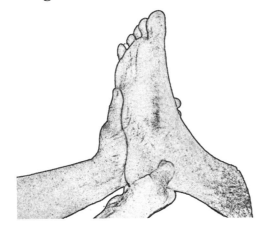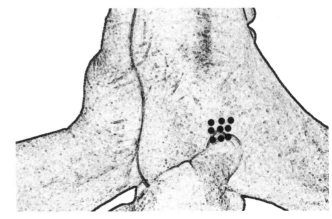

Helper Reflexes- **Adrenal** suppresses inflammation.

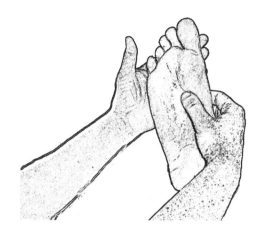
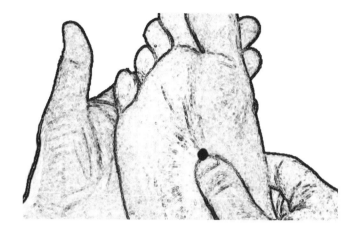

Ovaries helps to release estrogen and progesterone.

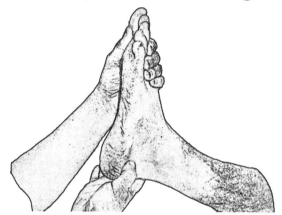
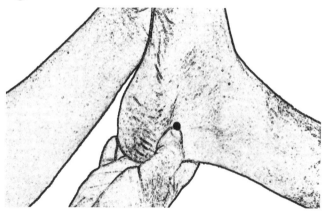

Thyroid helps with menstrual regularity.

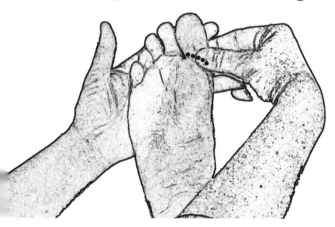
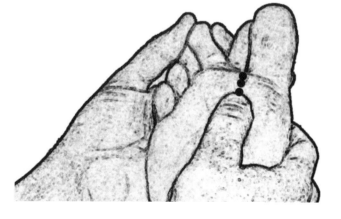

Solar plexus helps with relaxing the body.

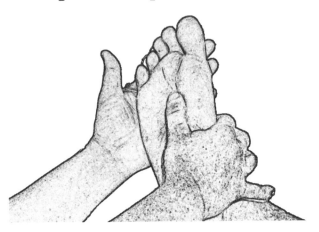
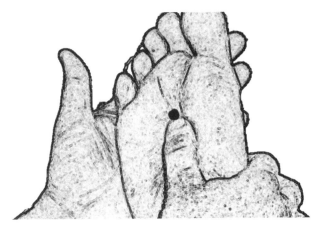

PMS- there are many reasons for PMS including progesterone deficiency, estrogen excess, hormonal imbalances, vitamin and mineral deficiency, and stress. A University did a test on 100 women that experienced PMS, and 75% were helped through reflexology.

Direct Reflex- Ovary helps to release progesterone.

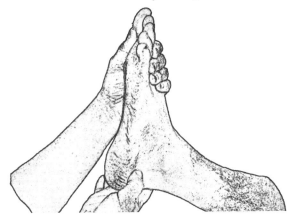
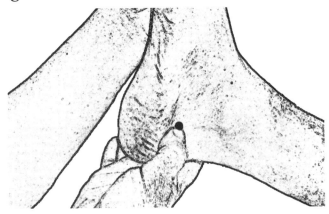

Helper Reflexes- Adrenal helps to release adrenaline for emotional stress.

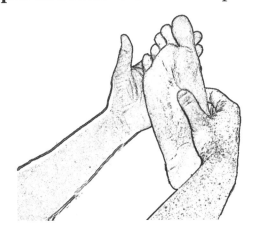
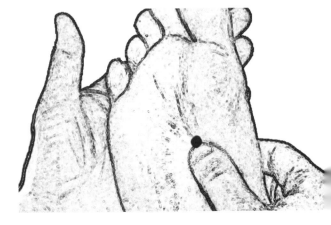

Hypothalamus helps to release hormones for emotions.

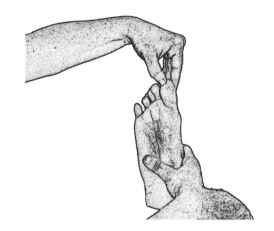 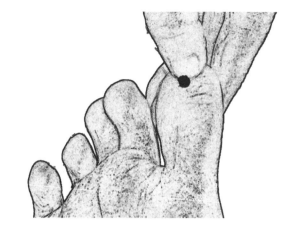

Thyroid regulates organ function.

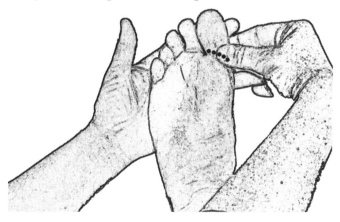 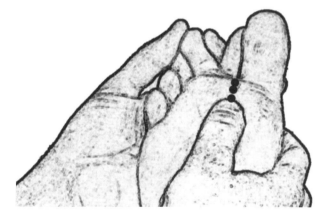

Solar plexus helps relieve stress and tension.

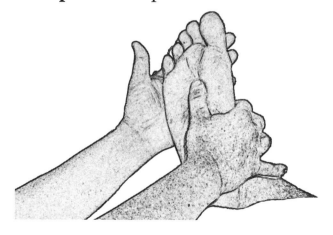 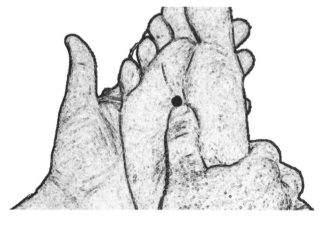

Pregnancy- conception occurs during ovulation as the egg enters the fallopian when the sperm fertilizes it.

Direct Reflex- Ovary helps to produce eggs.

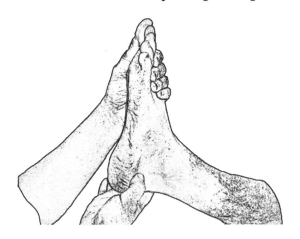 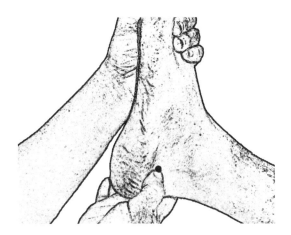

Helper Reflexes- Adrenal helps to release adrenaline for emotional stress.

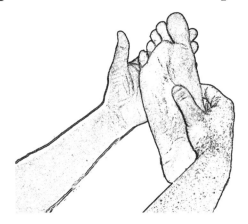 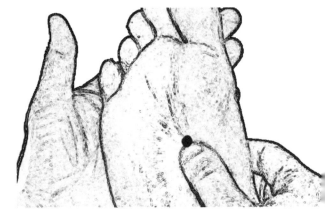

Hypothalamus /Pituitary helps to stimulate the ovary.

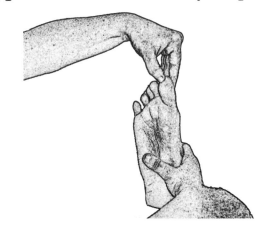 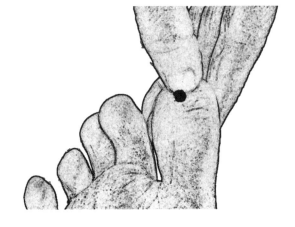

hyroid regulates organ function.

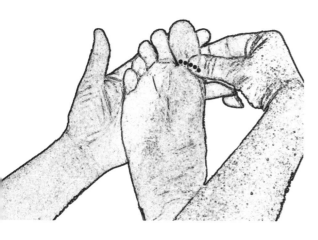 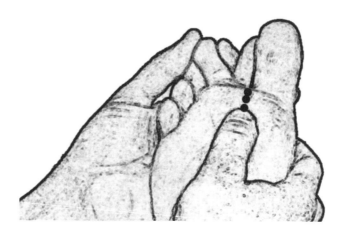

varian Cyst- is a fluid-filled sac in the ovary.
he University of California did a test on women with ovarian cyst. 62% of e women were helped through reflexology. The studied reported the cysts tually shrank.

rect Reflex- Ovary helps to break up the ovary.

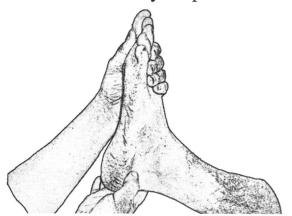 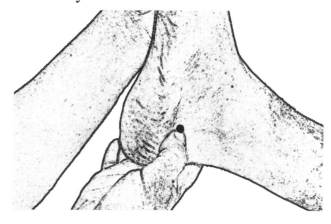

lper Reflexes- Adrenal it suppresses inflammation.

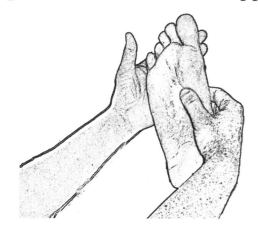 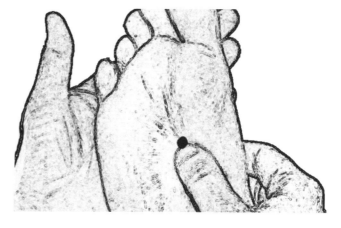

Hypothalamus / Pituitary helps with fluid retention.

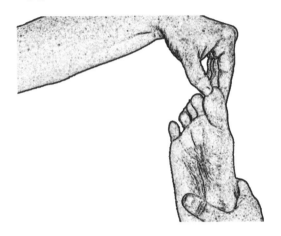 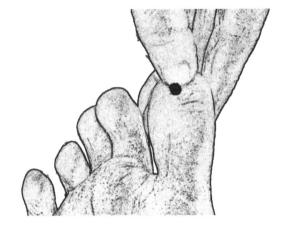

Thyroid helps to release thyroxine to regulate the organ.

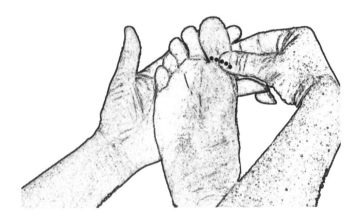 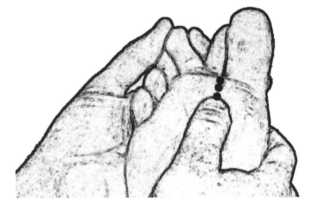

Cyst on the Breast- is a fluid-filled sac on the breast.

Direct Reflex- Breast helps to break up the cyst.

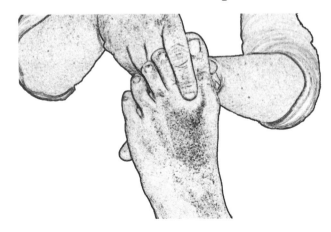 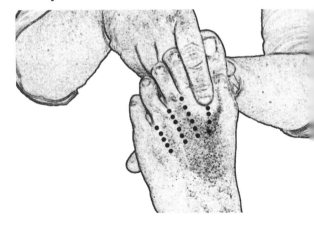

elper Reflexes- Adrenal suppresses inflammation.

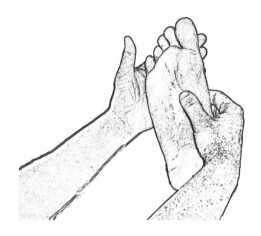
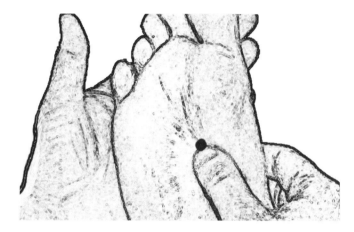

tuitary helps with fluid retention.

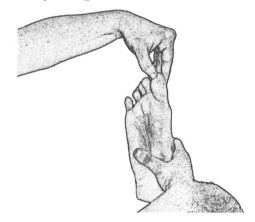
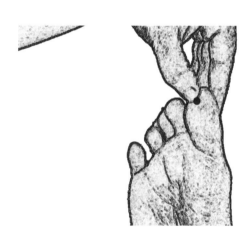

yroid releases thyroxine to regulate tissue in the breast.

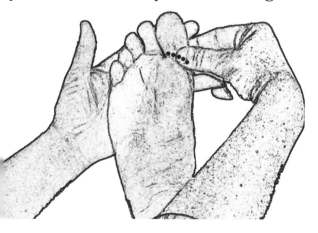
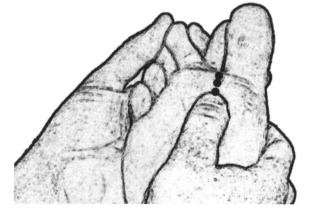

Uterine Fibroids are non-cancerous tumors of the uterus. They are attached to the uterus wall and are made up of fibrous tissue and muscle. It may cause heavy bleeding, pelvic discomfort and create pressure on other organs.

Direct reflex- Uterus- helps to break up the fibroids, you may feel this area to be lumpy like little bubbles.

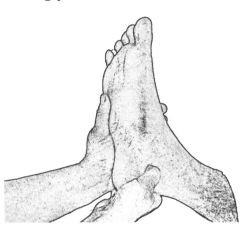
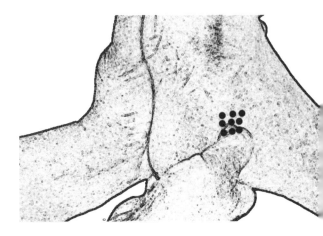

Helper Reflexes- Ovary helps to release estrogen and progesterone.

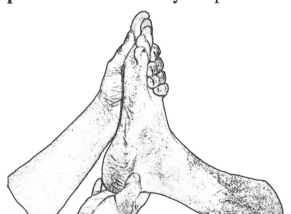
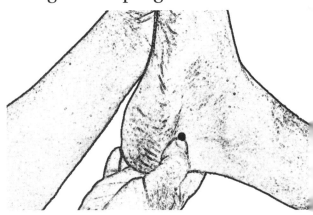

Pituitary this master gland helps with the ovaries function to release estrogen and progesterone.

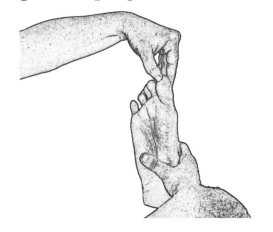
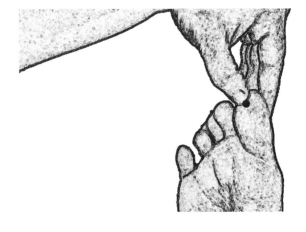

Male Reproductive Disorders and the Helper Reflex Areas

Enlarged Prostate Gland- an abnormal swelling of the tissues of the prostate, which causes difficulties with urinating.

Direct Reflex- Prostate helps to secrete the fluid part of the semen.

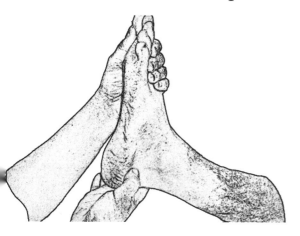
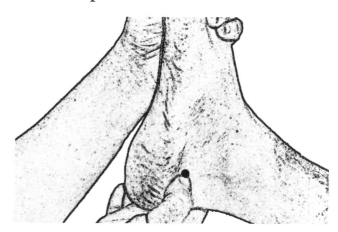

Helper Reflexes- Adrenal helps with releasing an Aldosterone hormone which controls the level of sodium excreted into the urine.

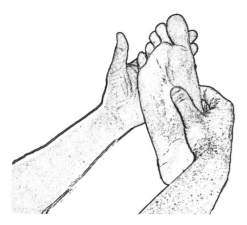
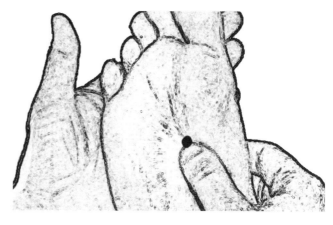

Bladder to strengthen.

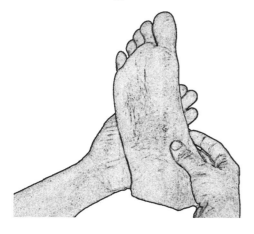
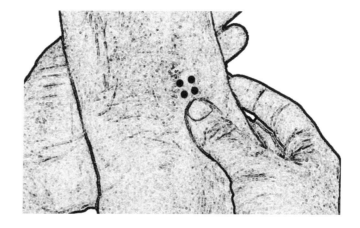

Chronic prostate area helps with reducing swelling.

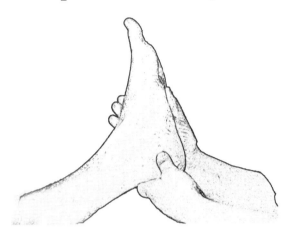 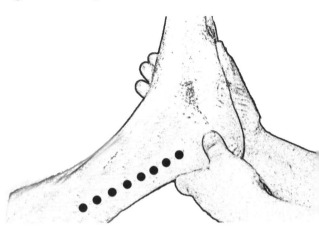

4th Lumbar to aid better blood and nerve supply.

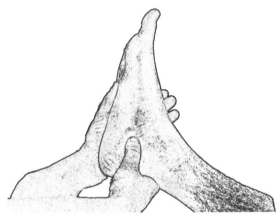 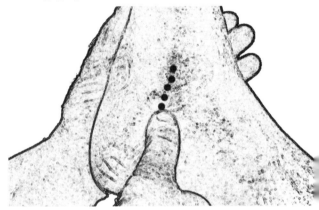

Impotence- failure to achieve or to maintain an erection.

Direct Reflex- Testes help to secrete testosterone.

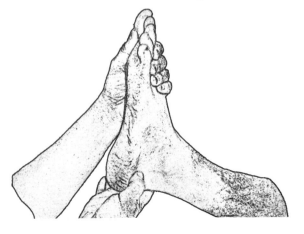 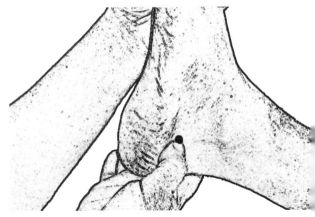

Helper Reflexes- Adrenal helps to release adrenaline for better blood flow to the muscle.

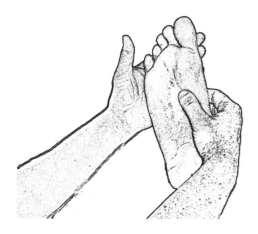
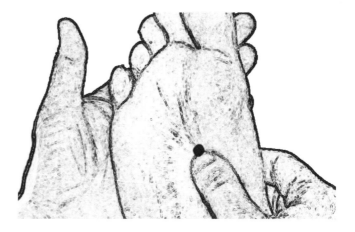

Hypothalamus/Pituitary helps the testes.

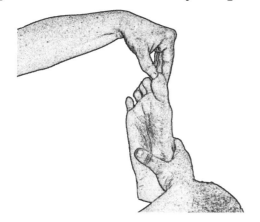
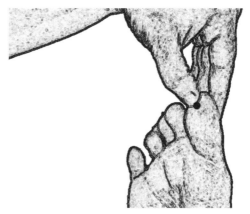

Lumbar to aid better blood and nerve supply.

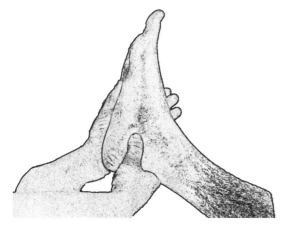
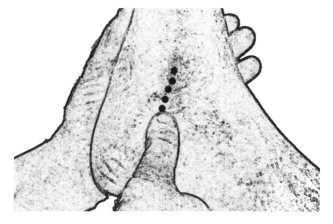

Infertility- when the testes do not produce sperm, or low sperm count.

Direct Reflex- Testes secretes testosterone.

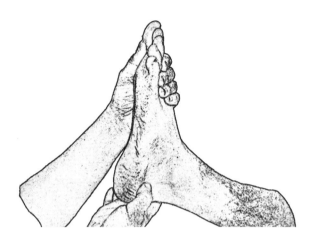 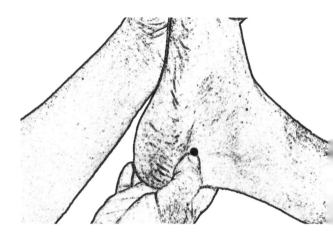

Helper Reflexes- Adrenal helps to release adrenaline for physical and emotional stress.

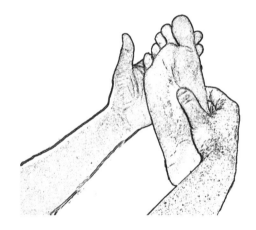 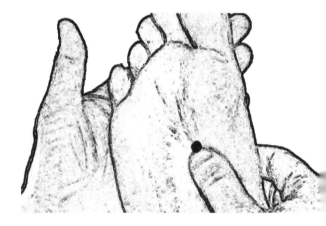

Hypothalamus helps with releasing hormones for expressions of emotions

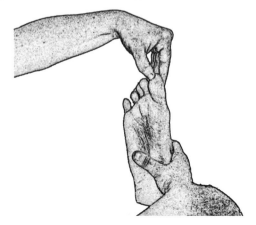 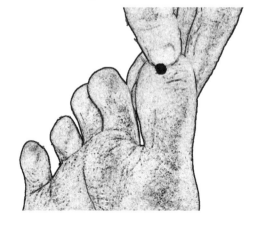

umbar to aid better blood and nerve supply.

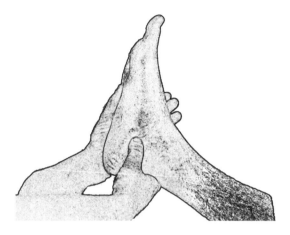 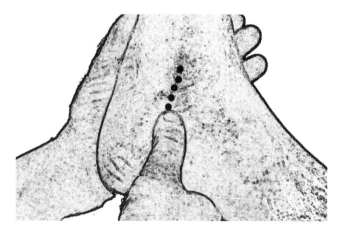

hyroid it influences the testes.

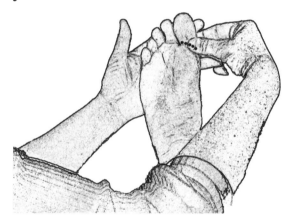 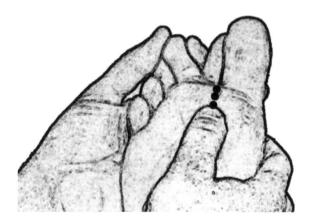

lar plexus helps for stress and tension.

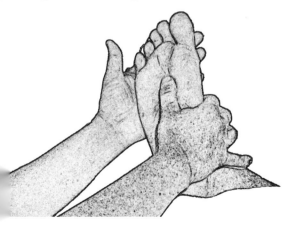 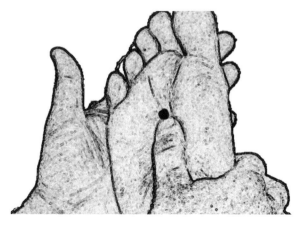

Quiz on the Reproductive System

1. What is the function of the uterus?
   A) to produce eggs and female hormones
   B) the development of the fetus take place here
   C) passageway for the egg

2. Where is the uterus reflex area located?
   A) lateral side between the ankle and heel
   B) top of the foot from ankle bone the ankle bone
   C) medial side between ankle bone and heel

3. What is the function of the ovary?
   A) passageway for the egg
   B) to produce eggs and female hormones
   C) the development of the fetus takes place here

4. Where is the ovary reflex area located?
   A) top of the foot from ankle bone to ankle bone
   B) lateral side between the ankle and heel
   C) medial side between ankle and heel

5. What is the function of the prostate?
   A) secretes the fluid part of of the semen
   B) produces sperm and the male hormone

6. Where is the prostate reflex area located?
   A) medial side between the ankle and the heel
   B) lateral side between the ankle and heel

7. What is the function of the testes?
   A) secretes the fluid part of the semen
   B) produces sperm and a male hormone

8. Where is the testes reflex area?
   A) medial side between the ankle and heel
   B) lateral side between the ankle and heel

* Answer key on page 325

15

The Skin

The Skin

The skin covering our entire body is the largest organ of the body. It weighs approximately six pounds in an adult. The skin regulates our body temperature, stores water, fat, vitamin D, and can transmit painful or pleasurable sensations. The soles of our feet and hands have thicker layers of skin. The skin is divided into three layers: epidermis, dermis, and the subcutaneous fat.

The **epidermis** is the outer layer of the skin that provides protection from the environment and stops foreign substances from invading our body.

The **dermis** is the middle layer, made up of blood vessels, lymph vessels, sweat glands, and hair follicles. The dermis has an important function of thermoregulation and supports the vascular network to supply the epidermis with nutrients.

The **subcutaneous fat** layer is responsible for insulation and shock absorbency.

The skin reflex areas are on both feet in Zone 5 on the lateral (outside) part of the foot. Thumb-walk these areas.

How to Work the Skin Organ Reflex Areas

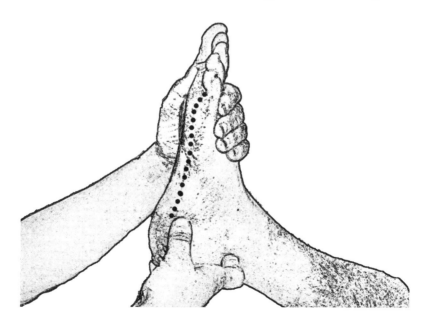

Locate the Reflex areas of the Largest Organ of the Body, the Skin

*Use colored pencils to draw in reflex areas

    A) Skin

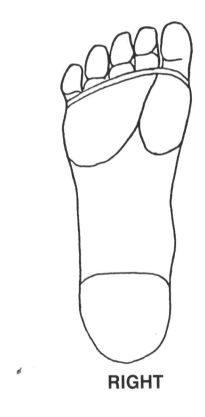

RIGHT

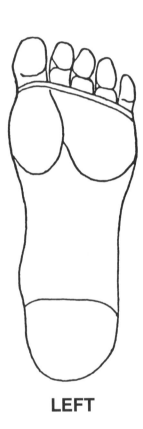

LEFT

Skin Disorders and the Helper Reflex Areas

Skin Disorders can be a result of body process, injuries, environment, hormone imbalance, germs, or fungus.

Direct Reflex- Endocrine glands helps for hormonal imbalances.

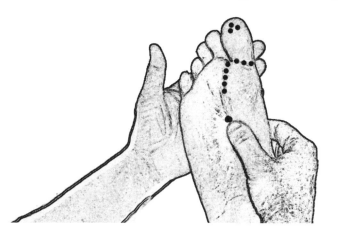
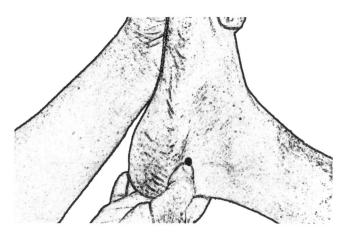

Helper Reflexes- Solar plexus for stress.

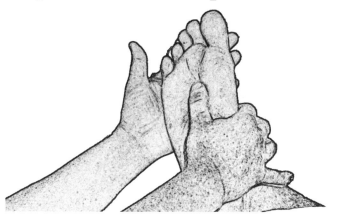
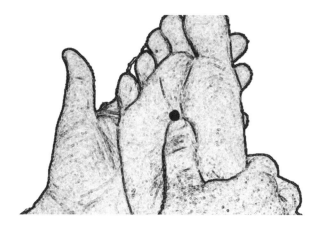

Liver to detoxify.

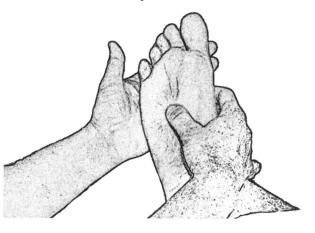
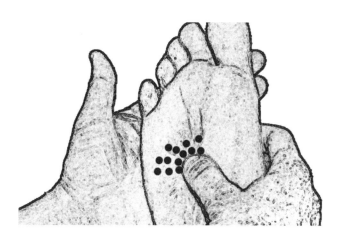

Large intestines to detoxify.

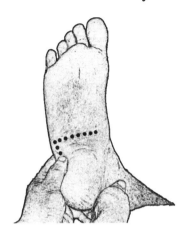
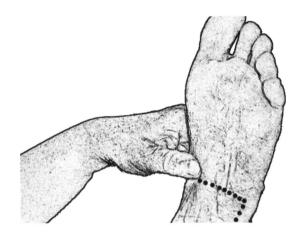

Acne is a common disorder, affecting mostly teenagers. When the hormone levels increases the skin may react. Bacteria on the skin is another cause which could produce pimples.

Direct Reflex- Endocrine glands helps for hormonal imbalances.

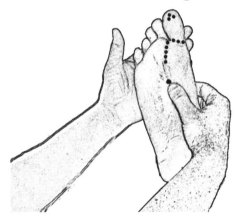
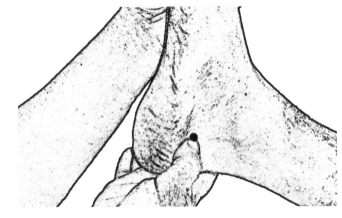

Helper Reflexes- Liver to detoxify.

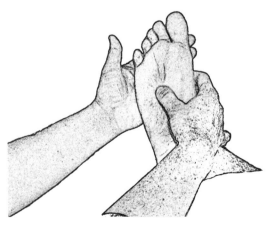
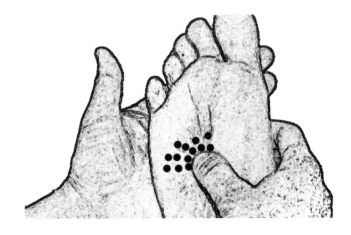

Kidneys to purify the blood.

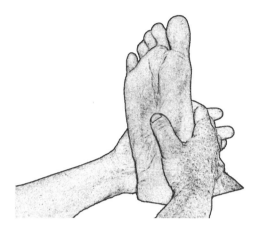
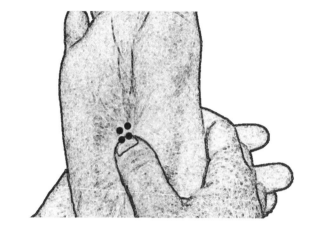

Large intestines to detoxify.

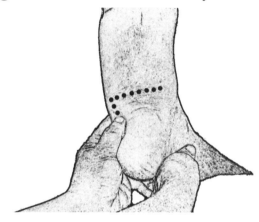
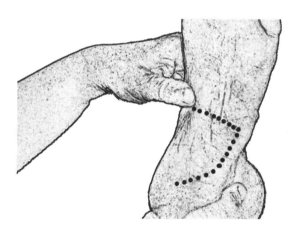

Eczema is very dry skin. It could be caused by an inherently sensitive skin, or an irritation from detergents, solvents, or oils, or an allergy to things such as cement or nickel.

Direct Reflex- Endocrine glands helps for skin conditions.

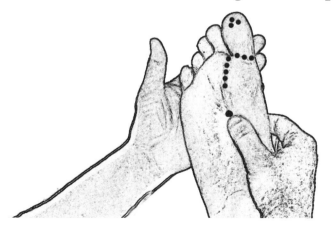
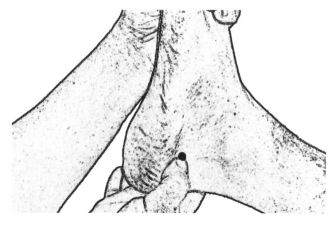

Helper Reflexes- **Large intestines** to detoxify.

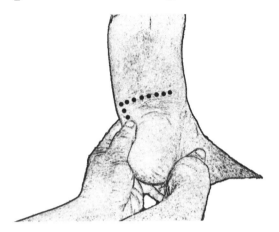
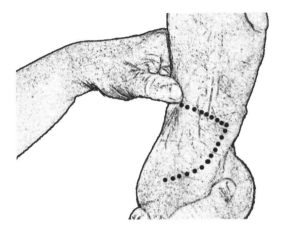

Liver to detoxify the harmful chemicals.

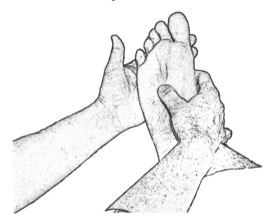
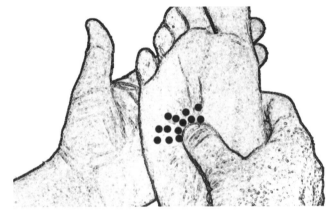

Kidney to purify the blood.

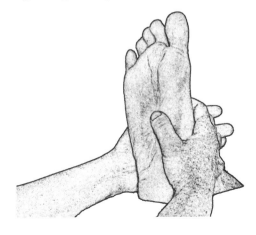
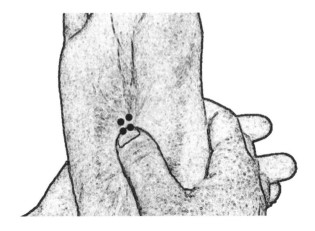

Solar plexus for stress.

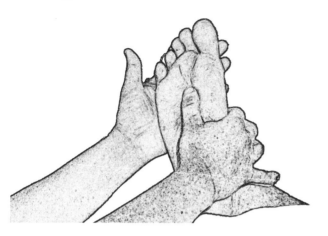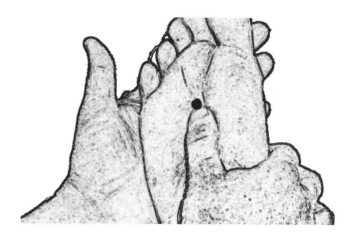

Psoriasis is an inflammatory skin disorder. It is thickened, red, scaly, patches appearing all over the skin and scalp.

Direct Reflex- Adrenal for inflammation.

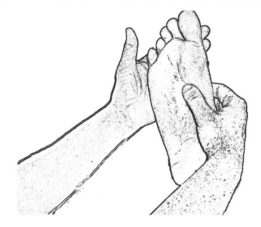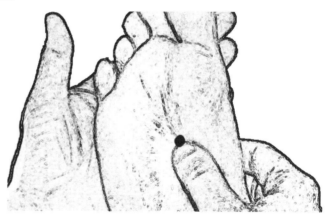

Solar plexus for stress.

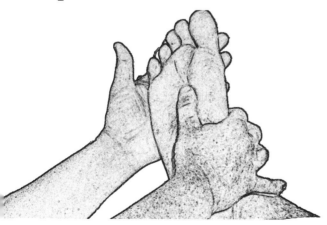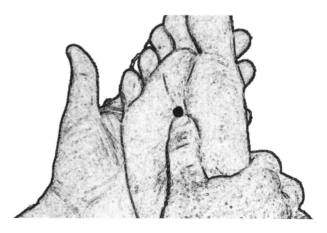

Helper Reflexes- Thyroid for skin conditions.

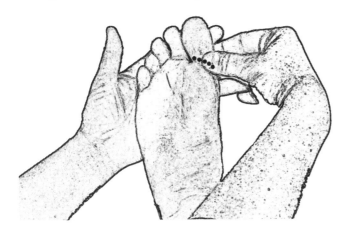 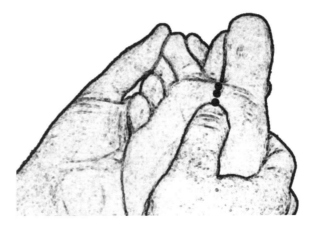

Large intestines to detoxify.

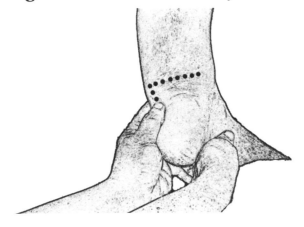 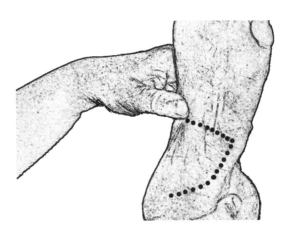

Kidneys to purify the blood.

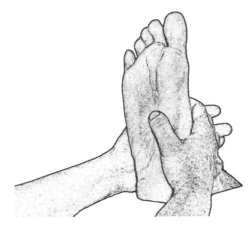 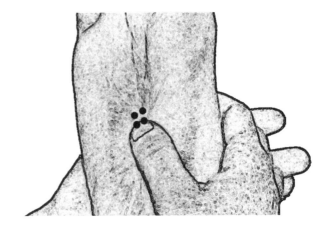

Tinea pedis (Athlete's foot) - is a fungus of the foot.

Quiz on the Skin Anatomy

1. Is the skin the largest organ of the body?
   A) Yes
   B) No

2. How many layers are in the skin?
   A) 4
   B) 3
   C) 2

3. Approximately how much does the skin weigh on an adult?
   A) 10 pounds
   B) 6 pounds
   C) 3 pounds

4. What layer is the epidermis?
   A) middle
   B) outer
   C) fat layer

5. What layer is the dermis?
   A) middle
   B) outer
   C) fat layer

6. Where is the skin reflex found on the feet?
   A) lateral part of the foot
   B) medial part of the foot
   C) heel line

* Answer key on page 325

Chapter **16** Foot Ailments

Pathologies of the Foot

Blisters - is a result of friction, blisters form to protect an area.

Bunion - (hallux valgus) hallux means great toe and valgus means deforming away from the mid-line of the body by a tendon, it is a deviation in the big toe joint.

Calluses - is located at the bottom of the foot, and is nothing more than a build-up of thick skin to protect a part of the body that is subjected to stress.

Claw toes - is when both interphalangeal joints are contracted.

Corns - (heloma) it is a thickened areas of the skin that appears between toes or side of the toes and on top of the toes.

Diabetic Neuropathy - is nerve damage from high blood sugars.

Gout - is a result of a build-up of uric acid in the blood and affects the great toe joint.

Hammer toes - is a contracture of the proximal joint.

Heel bursitis - is an inflammation of the heel.

Heel spurs - a calcium build-up on the calcaneous.

Ingrown toenails - is a piece of nail that grows into the side of the nail bed and causes discomfort.

Neuroma - is a pinched nerve that has erupted because of constant compression and irritation, either between the metatarsal heads, or at the base of the proximal phalanges.

Plantar fasciitis - is inflammation at the plantar (bottom) part of the foot.

Plantar warts - an internal virus infection that grows on the bottom foot. It is very contagious.

Post-tib tendonitis - is an inflammation of the tibial tendon.

Sesamoiditis - is inflammation of the sesamoids (two small bones at the first metatarsal. The tendons become inflamed.

Sprain - is trauma to the joint or injury to the ligaments.

Subluxation - a partial dislocation of the joint.

Foot Ailments

A Bunion- is a misaligned great toe joint which can be swollen. A bunion often can causes pain and swelling. The pain is from tight fitting shoes.

Relieve the pain by thumb or finger-walking around the bunion, then work over the bunion gradually adding pressure.

Diabetic Foot Problem- Neuropathy- is nerve damage from high blood sugars. Pain or numbness in the legs and feet are common complaints.

Reflexology helps to get better blood flow to all extremities and some of my clients notice a reduction of pain in their feet and legs. Some of them can feel their feet again! Thumb-walk every part of their feet.

Heel Spurs- are growths of bone on the bottom part of the heel bone. Heel spurs occur when the plantar tendon pulls at its attachment to the heel bone. This can later calcify to form a spur.

Thumb-walk the entire calcaneous (heel). It will be painful, so go lightly to begin with, and gradually add pressure. Work the pain out.

Morton's Neuroma- are large benign growths of nerves, mostly common between the third and fourth toes. They are cause by tissue rubbing against nerves which swells.

To relieve pain and discomfort thumb-walk the area and gradually add pressure.

Plantar Fasciitis- is inflammation at the bottom of the foot. Plantar Fascia is a ligament-like band running from the heel to the pad of the foot. This band pulls on the heel bone, raising the arch of the foot as it pushes off the ground so that it becomes strained. The fascia swells and its tiny fibers begin to fray causing fasciitis.

To relieve pain and discomfort thumb-walk all Zones from heel line to the diaphragm line. You may feel this area to be lumpy, work the lumps out.

Sesamoiditis- is an inflammation of the sesamoid (two small bones at the first metatarsal) at the ball-of-the-foot, causing extreme pain. The tendons around the bones become inflamed as well. It is caused by repetitive pressure on the ball of the foot, such as running or dancing.

To relieve pain and discomfort. With your holding hand spread the toes between Zones 1-2, 2-3, 3-4, 4-5. With your working hand thumb-walk between all metatarsal. You may feel this area to be full of inflammation. Work it out.

Post-Tib Tendonitis- is an inflammation of the tibial tendon. Over use of this tendon may get it inflamed.

To relieve the pain and discomfort, pull great toe back and run your finger along Zone 1 to find the tibial tendon. Thumb-walk along each side of it, not directly on it.

Flat Feet- is when the arch has collapsed.

In some cases it may cause Plantar Fasciitis. Thumb-walk all zones from the heel line to the diaphragm line.

How to Work Foot Ailments

To work a **bunion** use finger-walking around the bunion, then go over it several times from different directions, gradually adding pressure.

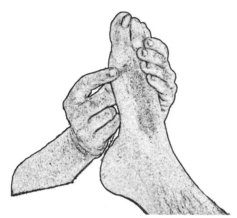
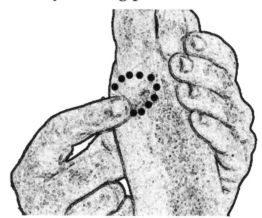

To work a **heel spur** use the thumb-walking around it, then over it several times to help with the inflammation around it. It is painful while working this area, but if the client can stand it they benefit so much. Thumb-walk the whole calcaneous (heel).

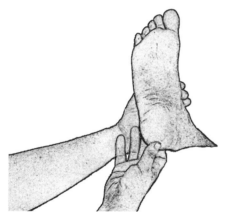
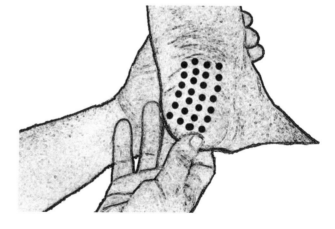

To work the **Sesamoiditis area**, thumb-walk between metatarsals 1 and 2, spread the toes to thumb-walk up. In many clients I have felt inflammation between all the metatarsals. Spread toes and thumb-walk up.

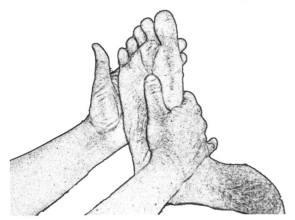
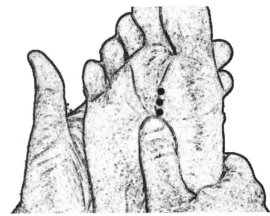

To work the **post-tib tendonitis**, pull the great toe back and the tendon will be visible, thumb-walk each side of the tendon, not directly on the tendon.

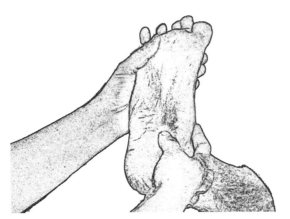
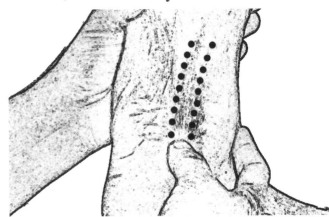

To work the **Morton's Neuroma**, thumb-walk the area that is affected. It relieves the pain instantly.

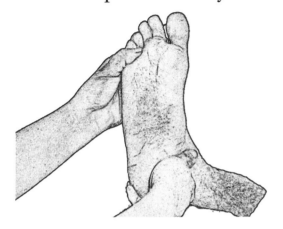 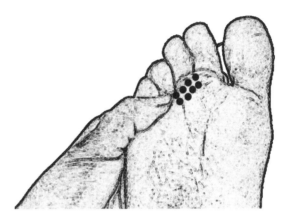

To work the **Plantar Fasciitis**, thumb-walk starting from the heel line up to the diaphragm line. Thumb-walk all the zones. This area could be lumpy, so keep working and you can usually smooth it out.

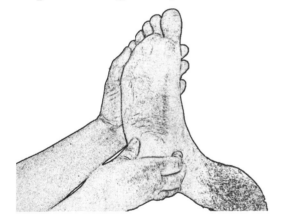 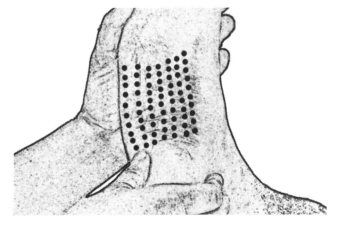

To work **heel bursitis**, thumb-walk across the entire heel this will be painful, but work out the lumps these are bursa sacs. The pain will be eliminated.

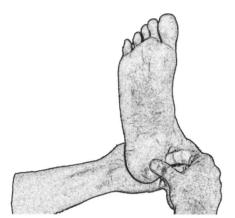 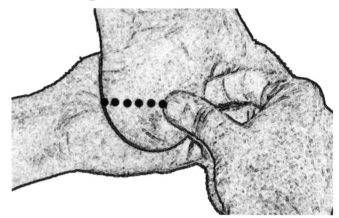

Chapter 17

Sample Reflexology Session

Steps in Giving a Reflexology Session

1) Make sure you file your nails and wash your hands.

2) Have client fill out client history form, then make a chart for them (draw a pair of feet). Mark the sensitivity spots and foot problem areas when you are finished with the session.

3) Greet the feet and check for bruises, bunion, calluses, corns, cuts, fungus, and warts. If there are any, make your client aware of them. On your chart mark where the problem areas are.

4) If it is the clients first session, explain the concepts of reflexology.

5) *** Rule of Thumb: Keep your eye on the clients face and watch for expressions of pain, and communicate with your client, if you feel they are in pain let off of the pressure and gradually work up to moderate pressure.**

6) I start on the right foot with relaxing techniques. Before going on to the left foot, I thoroughly work all reflexes on the right foot.

7) Thumb-walk the spinal reflexes (from the inside of the foot starting from just below the heel line to almost to the top of the toes). Thumb-press the solar plexus.

8) Finger-rock the brain reflexes (all the tips of toes).

9) Thumb-walk down on the head and sinuses reflexes (all the toes).

10) Thumb-press the pituitary and hypothalamus (great toe).

11) Thumb-walk across the T.M.J./jaw reflexes (it is about three-quarters down on the great toe).

12) Thumb-walk across the thyroid and neck reflexes (great toe line) and thumb-walk for the muscle on the side of the neck (inside of the grea toe).

13) Thumb-walk the ear and eye reflexes (starting from outside on the to line thumb-walk in towards the great toe.)

14) Finger-walk breast/chest reflexes (make a fist, push on ball of the foo to spread the metatarsals, and finger-walk down between the metatarsals).

15) Thumb-walk the thyroid/bronchial, esophagus, heart, lung, shoulder arm, and wrist reflexes (work everything between the toe line and diaphragm line.)

16) Do some relaxing techniques.

17 A) Thumb-walk all reflexes between diaphragm line to the waistline. On the right foot it is the liver/gallbladder, kidney, adrenal, duodenum, and the head of the pancreas.

17 B) On the left foot the reflexes are stomach, spleen, adrenal, kidney and pancreas.

18 A) Thumb-press the ileocecal valve in zone 5 at the heel line. Thumb walk up the ascending colon in zone 5 and across 4-1 zones for the transverse colon just below the waistline.

18 B) On the left foot thumb-walk across zones 1-4 for the transverse colon just below the waistline and down the descending colon in zor 5. Thumb-press the sigmoid flexure in zone 4 just past the heel line.

19) Thumb-walk the small intestines zones 1-4 between the waist line ar heel line.

20) Thumb-walk across the sciatic nerve between the heel line and back of the heel.

21) Finger-walk the hip, knee, and leg reflexes. They are located on the lateral (outside) side of the foot in the triangle area between the cuboid and calcaneous (heel). If the hip,knee, and leg has chronic pain thumb or finger-walk down the lateral side of the leg to the talus (ankle bone)

22) Thumb-press the ovary/testes, reflex is located on the lateral (outside) part of the foot between the talus (ankle bone) and calcaneous (heel). Thumb-press the uterus/prostate, reflex is located on the medial (inside) part of the foot between the talus (ankle) and calcaneous (heel).

23) Finger-walk the fallopian tubes/lymphatic system on the dorsal (top) of the foot from talus to talus (ankle bone).

24) Go back over any sensitive areas.

25) Finish off with relaxation techniques and go to the left foot and start this process again!

26) Let your client know you will be calling them for a follow-up.

27) Finish filling the paper work out, while they relax.

Stretching your Hands between Clients to avoid Carpal Tunnel Syndrome

- Stay aware of your posture.

- Do shoulder rolls and shrugs.

- Shake out tension in hands and fingers.

- Shake out wrists and arms. Let your arms dangle from your shoulders and shake out.

- Wrist Rotation- make a fist and rotate your entire hand (from the wrist) in one direction. Repeat 15 times. Switch directions and repeat 15 times. Then, release your hands, and with fingers extended, do the same rotations. Repeat with the other hand.

- Hand Stretch- Make a fist, then extend your fingers as far apart as possible. Hold for about 10 seconds. Relax. Repeat 5-10 times. Repeat with other hand.

- Limbering Up- Massage the inside and outside of the hands. Grasp fingers and gently bend back at the wrist. Hold for 5 seconds. Gently pull thumb down and back until you feel the stretch. Hold for 5 seconds. Repeat with other hand.

* Keep you body and wrists relaxed while working on your clients

Chapter 18

Marketing, Client History Forms, and Documenting Charts

How to Market Yourself

The best way I have found to market Reflexology is to contact your local paper and an independent newspaper. Talk to a writer and offer her/him a session with reflexology. They are always interested in writing articles about different topics. Then you can advertise your business following the article. With my experiences, advertising without the article could be a waste of money because most people do not know what reflexology is so you need to educate them!

Another way to market yourself is setting up a booth at a health fair. Have your brochures and business cards ready and give demonstrations.

Give speeches at women's clubs, nursing home and independent Living facilities. Word of mouth is always your best advertising. Be professional, dress appropriately, be enthusiastic, compassionate, and always be friendly!!

Sample Client History Form

Name _____

Address _____

City _____ State _____ Zip _____

Hm. Phone _____ Bus. Phone _____

How would you rate your health? ❑Excellent ❑Good ❑Fair ❑Poor

Doctor's care? ❑Yes ❑No

Are you on medication? ❑Yes ❑No

List the medication _____

Are you receiving any other therapies? _____

Is this your first reflexology session? _____

Any present illnesses? _____

Any past surgeries? _____

Any foot injuries? _____

If you have a serious illness you should speak to your doctor before embarking on this program of reflexology. Tell him/her what you plan on doing. Do not stop or adjust medications before you speak with your doctor.

Sample Client History Form
Documenting Your Sessions

Name _____

Address _____

City _____ State: ____ Zip: _____

Hm. Phone _____ Bus. Phone _____

Mark on the feet if there are any foot problems or injuries.

Mark on the feet where the sensitivity spots are, label 1-4 with 1 as slightly uncomfortable and 4 as intense pain.

RIGHT   **LEFT**

RIGHT OUTSIDE

TOP RIGHT   **TOP LEFT**

LEFT OUTSIDE

On the back of this form write your comments on your client. Keep records and document each time.

19

Reflexology Foot Charts

RIGHT FOOT

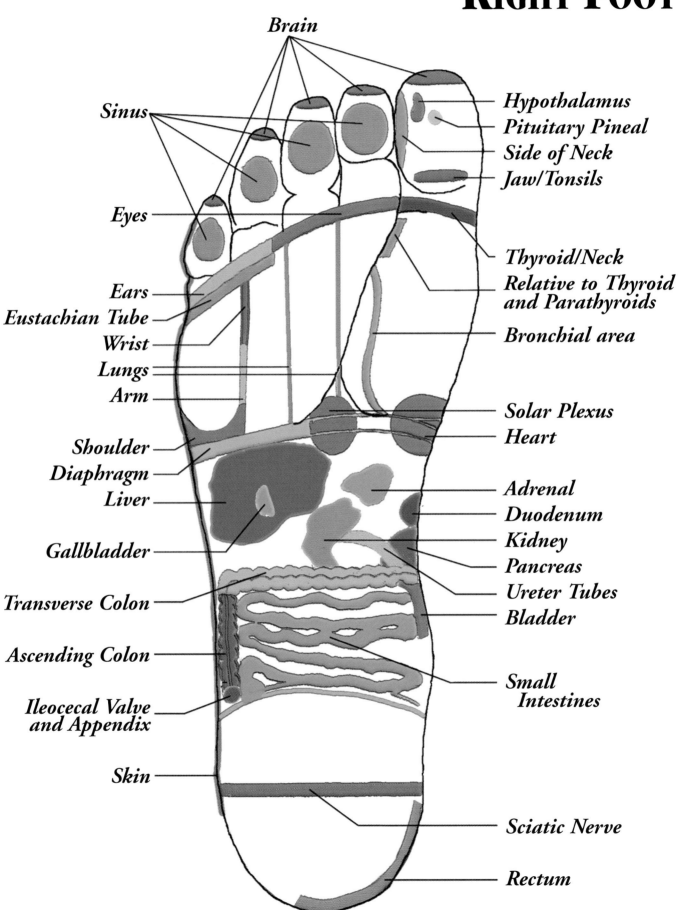

Brain

Sinus

Hypothalamus
Pituitary Pineal
Side of Neck
Jaw/Tonsils

Eyes

Thyroid/Neck
Relative to Thyroid
and Parathyroids

Ears
Eustachian Tube
Wrist
Lungs
Arm

Bronchial area

Solar Plexus
Heart

Shoulder
Diaphragm
Liver

Adrenal
Duodenum
Kidney
Pancreas
Ureter Tubes

Gallbladder

Transverse Colon

Bladder

Ascending Colon

Ileocecal Valve
and Appendix

Small
Intestines

Skin

Sciatic Nerve

Rectum

LEFT FOOT

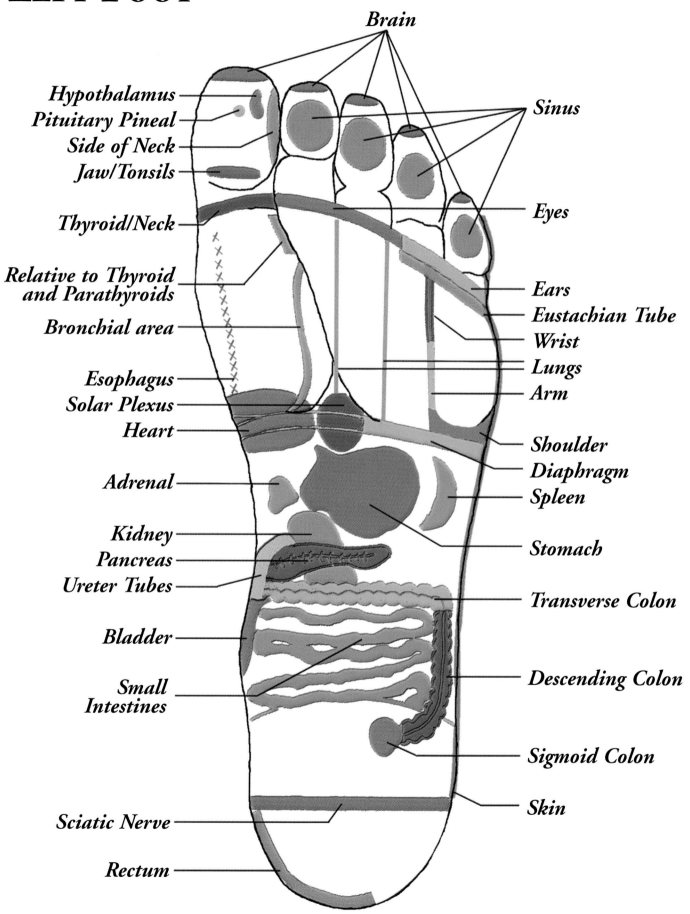

Brain

Hypothalamus
Pituitary Pineal
Side of Neck
Jaw/Tonsils

Sinus

Thyroid/Neck

Eyes

Relative to Thyroid
and Parathyroids

Bronchial area

Ears
Eustachian Tube
Wrist
Lungs
Arm

Esophagus
Solar Plexus
Heart

Shoulder
Diaphragm
Spleen

Adrenal

Kidney
Pancreas
Ureter Tubes

Stomach

Transverse Colon

Bladder

Small
Intestines

Descending Colon

Sigmoid Colon

Skin

Sciatic Nerve

Rectum

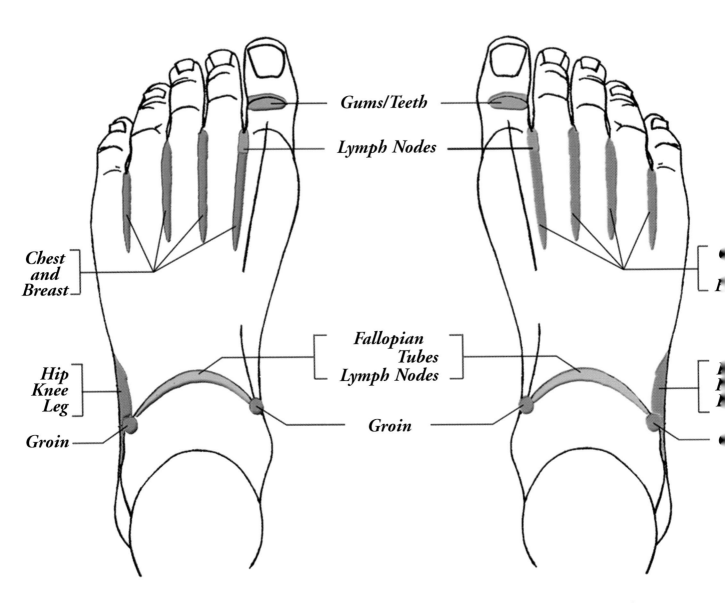

TOP LEFT

TOP RIGHT

Gums/Teeth

Lymph Nodes

Chest
and
Breast

Fallopian
Tubes
Lymph Nodes

Hip
Knee
Leg

Groin

Groin

INSIDE

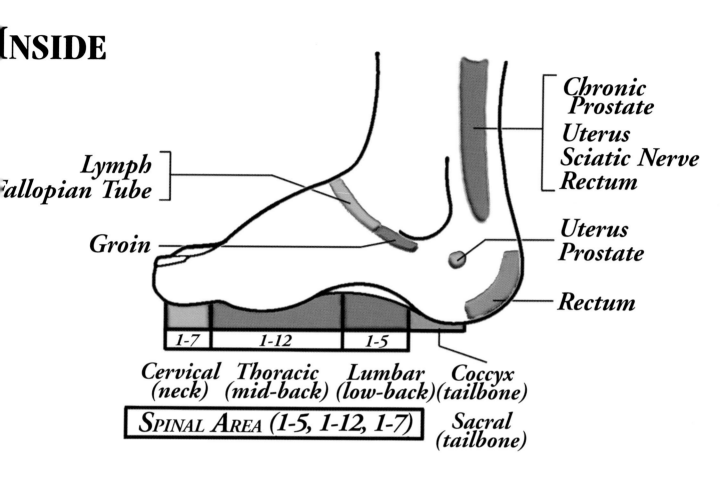

Lymph
Fallopian Tube

Groin

Chronic
Prostate
Uterus
Sciatic Nerve
Rectum

Uterus
Prostate

Rectum

| 1-7 | 1-12 | 1-5 |

Cervical   Thoracic   Lumbar   Coccyx
(neck)   (mid-back) (low-back)(tailbone)

SPINAL AREA (1-5, 1-12, 1-7)   Sacral
(tailbone)

OUTSIDE

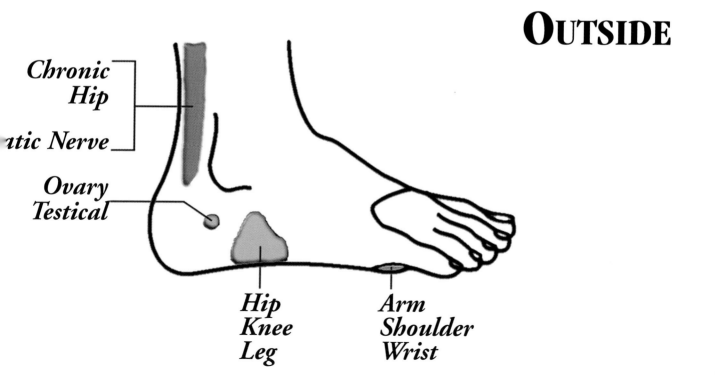

Chronic
Hip

Sciatic Nerve

Ovary
Testical

Hip
Knee
Leg

Arm
Shoulder
Wrist

Answer Key to the Quizzes

Quiz on Anatomy of the foot, guidelines, and the zones

1. C	6. B
2. A	7. B
3. C	8. A
4. A	9. B
5. C	10. C

Quiz on the Central Nervous System

1. A	6. C
2. C	7. B
3. B	8. B
4. C	9. A
5. B	10. A

Quiz on the Sense Organs

1. B	5. B
2. A	6. B
3. A	7. B
4. B	8. B

Quiz on the Endocrine System

1. B	6. B
2. C	7. A
3. B	8. A
4. A	9. B
5. B	10. C

Quiz on the Circulatory System

1. C	4. A
2. B	5. A
3. A	6. C

Quiz on the Digestive System

1. A	6. A
2. A	7. A
3. B	8. A
4. C	9. A
5. A	

Quiz on the Urinary System

1. B	4. B
2. A	5. C
3. A	6. B

Quiz on the Respiratory System

1. A	5. A
2. C	6. B
3. A	7. C
4. B	8. B

Quiz on the Lymphatic System

1. A	4. B
2. A	5. B
3. B	6. A

Quiz on the Hip, Knee, Shoulder, Elbow, and Wrist

1. C	5. A
2. B	6. A
3. B	7. B
4. C	8. A

Quiz on the Reproductive System

1. B	5. A
2. C	6. A
3. B	7. B
4. B	8. B

Quiz in the Skin Anatomy

1. A	4. B
2. B	5. A
3. B	6. A

Index

A

Abduction - 27, 30
Adduction - 27-30
Acne - 286
ADD - 13, 14, 115
AD/HD - 13, 14, 116
Adrenal - 103, 104, 108, 112, 117
Allergies - 213
Alveoli - 207, 208
Angina Pectoris - 134
Anemia - 233
Answer Key to the Quizzes - 325
Anterior - 26
Anvil - 83, 84
Aortic Valve - 129, 130
Arteries - 130
Arterioles - 130
Ascending Colon - 148, 156
Asthma - 214, 215
Athlete's Feet - 8, 290
Atrial Fibrillation - 136, 137
Atrium - 129, 130
Auricle - 83, 84

B

Bedwetting - 192
Bells Palsy - 64
Bladder - 187, 188, 191
Blood Vessels - 130
Brain - 51, 52, 53, 54, 60
Breast - 256, 261
Bronchial Tubes - 207, 208, 211
Bronchi - 206, 208
Bronchitis - 216
Bruises - 8
Bunion - 295, 297, 299

C

Calcaneus - 21, 22, 24
Cancer - 16, 17
Capillaries - 130
Carpal Tunnel - 249-250
Cataracts - 94
Central Nervous System - 51, 54, 55
Cerebellum - 51, 52
Cerebrum - 51, 52
Cervical - 53, 62
Choroid - 81, 82
Chronic Prostate - 262, 275
Chronic Uterus - 262

Coccyx - 53, 55, 61
Cochlea - 83, 84
Conjunctiva - 81, 82
Constipation - 160
Cornea - 81, 82
Corticotropin - 103
Crohn's Disease - 162, 163
Cuboid - 21, 22
Cuneiforms - 21, 22
Cyst on breast - 272, 273
Cystitis - 193-194

D

Dermis - 283
Descending Colon - 157
Diabetes - 168, 169
Diagnose - 8
Diaphragm - 207, 208, 212
Diarrhea - 165
Digestive System - 147
Distal - 21, 22, 26
Diverticulosis - 170
Dorsal - 26
Dorsiflexion - 27, 31
Duodenum - 148, 150, 154

E

Ear Canal - 83, 84
Ear Drum - 83, 84
Ear Infection - 88
Ear Reflex - 87
Eczema - 287, 288
Elbow - 241, 242, 247
Emphysema - 218, 219
Endocrine Glands - 103, 112
Endocrine System - 103, 108, 112
Enlarged Prostate - 275
Epidermis - 283
Esophagus - 147, 154
Eustachian Tube - 83, 84
Eversion - 27, 31
Eyes - 81, 82

F

Fallopian Tubes - 256, 261
Finger-walking - 39
Finger-rocking - 40
Foot Stimulating - 45

G

Gallbladder - 149-158
Gallstones - 172
Glaucoma - 95
Growth Disorders - 120
Guidelines - 32

H

Hammer - 83, 84
Headache - 65
Heart - 129, 130
Heart Attack - 139
Heartburn - 173
Heel Spurs - 295, 297, 299
Hemorrhoids - 175
Herniated Disc - 67
Hip - 241-243
Hook-back - 40
Hot Flashes - 263
Hypertension - 121
Hyperthyroidism - 123
Hypoglycemia - 176
Hypothalamus - 104, 108
Hypothyroidism - 124

I

Ileocecal Valve - 148-155
Immune System - 234
Impotence - 276
Incontinence - 194
Infertility - 278
Ingrown Toenail - 8
Inversion - 27, 31
Iris - 81, 82
Irritable Bowel - 177
Islands of Langerhans - 106, 112, 149

J

Jaw - 68

K

Kidney - 187, 188, 191
Kidney Stones - 196
Knee - 241, 243, 246

Index

L

Large Intestines - 148, 150, 156, 157
Lateral - 26
Lens - 81, 82
Liver - 149, 150, 158
Lumbar - 53, 55, 61
Lungs - 205, 208, 212
Lymph Nodes - 227, 228, 231, 232
Lymphatic System - 227, 228, 232
Lymphoedema - 235
Lymphoma - 235

M

Macula - 82
Macular Degeneration - 96
Medial - 26
Medulla Oblongata - 52
Menopause - 265
Menstrual Cramping - 266
Metatarsal - 21, 22
Migraine - 68
Mitral Valve - 129-130
Morning Sickness - 179
Morton's Neuroma - 295, 297, 301
Motion Sickness - 180
Multiple Sclerosis - 69

N

Nausea - 181
Navicular - 21, 22
Nephritis - 199
Neuropathy - 297
Nose - 205, 208

O

Optic Nerve - 82
Ovarian Cyst - 271
Ovary - 255, 262

P

Palmar - 26
Pancreas - 149, 150, 159
Paralysis - 71
Parathyroid - 106, 108, 114
Parkinson's Disease - 72
Pericarditis - 141
Phalanges - 21, 22

Pharynx - 206, 208
Pineal Gland - 104
Pituitary - 105
Plantar - 22, 26
Plantar Fasciitis - 296, 298, 301
Plantar Flexion - 27, 31
Pneumonia - 219
Posterior - 26
PMS - 268
Pregnancy - 18, 270
Pronation - 27, 29
Prostate - 257, 262, 275
Proximal - 22, 26
Psoriasis - 289
Pulmonary Valve - 129, 130
Pupil - 81, 82

Q

R

Raynaud's disease - 235
Rectum - 153
Referral Area - 35, 249, 250
Reproductive System - 255
Respiratory System - 205
Retina - 82
Retinopathy - 98

S

Sacral - 53, 55, 61
Sacrum - 53, 55, 61
Sciatic Nerve - 56
Sciatica - 56
Sclera - 81-82
Semicircular Canals - 83, 84
Sense Organs - 81, 82
Sesamoid Bones - 21, 22
Shortness of Breath - 222
Shoulder - 241, 242, 247
Sigmoid Flexure - 149, 150, 157
Sinuses - 205, 206, 208, 211
Sinusitis - 221
Skin - 283
Small Intestines - 148, 150, 155
Solar Plexus - 56, 60
Spinal Cord - 52, 53, 54, 55
Spleen - 228
Sprained Ankle - 250
Stirrup - 83, 84
Stomach - 147, 150, 158
Strained Ankle - 250

Stroke - 74
Superficial - 26
Supination - 27, 29

T

Talus - 21, 22
Tennis Elbow - 251
Testes - 107, 108, 257
Thoracic - 53, 54, 55, 62
Thumb-walking - 39
Thumb-press - 40
Thymus - 227, 228
Thyroid - 105, 108
Tinnitus - 90
Tonsils - 227, 228, 231
Tonsillitis - 236
TMJ - 68
Trachea - 206
Transverse Colon - 156
Tricuspid Valve - 129, 130

U

Ulcer - 182
Ureter Tubes - 187, 188, 191
Uterus - 255, 262
Uterine Fibroids - 274
Urethra - 188
Urinary System - 187, 188

V

Veins - 130
Ventricle - 129, 130
Venules - 130
Vena Cava - 130
Vertigo - 92
Vestibule - 83, 84
Vitreous - 81, 82

W

Whiplash - 75
Wrist - 242, 247

X

Y

Z

Zones - 33

Order Information

Give the gift of
Master The Healing Art of Foot Reflexology
to your family, friends, and colleagues.

ORDER HERE

❏YES, I want_____copies of Master the Healing Art of Foot Reflexology (#9719437) for $34.95 each.

❏YES, I am interested in having Susan Watson speak or give a seminar to my company, association,school, or organization. Please send me the information.

Include $3.95 shipping and handling,
and $1.95 shipping, for each additional book.
Add applicable sales tax.
Canadian must include payment in US funds, with 7% GST added.

Payment must accompany orders. Allow 3-4 weeks for delivery.

My check or money order for $_____ is enclosed.

Name_____

Organization_____

Address _____

City_____ State ____ Zip _____

Phone (___) _____ E-mail_____

Make your check or money order payable and send to:
Susan Watson
PO Box 623
Durand IL 61024-0623
www.thumbwalking.com